YOGA FOR BENDY PEOPLE

YOGA FOR BENDY PEOPLE

OPTIMIZING THE BENEFITS OF YOGA FOR HYPERMOBILITY

LIBBY HINSLEY, PT, DPT, C-IAYT

NDP

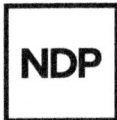

NEW DEGREE PRESS

YOGA FOR BENDY PEOPLE

Optimizing the Benefits of Yoga for Hypermobility

ISBN   979-8-88504-118-8   *Paperback*

             979-8-88504-746-3   *Kindle Ebook*

             979-8-88504-225-3   *Ebook*

For my spectacular daughters, Clementine and Marigold, who inspire me every day to be the best version of myself I can be.

And for all my fellow zebras out there—
I see you, and I celebrate you!

Disclaimer

This book is not intended to provide a diagnosis or treatment for Hypermobility Spectrum Disorder (HSD), Hypermobile Ehlers-Danlos Syndrome (hEDS), or any other condition, and it does not replace evaluation and treatment of a qualified healthcare professional. Please consult your doctor before undertaking any exercise program.

Contents

———

Foreword by Jill Miller

———

It all started innocently enough, my obsession with stretching.

I wanted to try out for the Flag Girls Team in seventh grade at Capshaw Junior High in Santa Fe. I was a young seventh-grader, a full year younger than all my peers. My twelve-year-old body was excessively lean due to my unchecked anorexia. The summer prior to seventh grade, I had discovered aerobics classes with my stepmother. It melted off thirty-five pounds of elementary school baby fat, and I was finally free from being teased.

To make the Flag Girls Team, I needed to be able to do cartwheels and drop into the splits, or so I thought. I had the cartwheel part, but splits were out of my range.

The road to splits could be conquered, I thought, with my mom's Raquel Welch Yoga video. I had dabbled with it before and knew how painful stretching could be. Stretching had always hurt because I wasn't used to moving. I had been a completely sedentary child. I was a reader and doll player, the thick-glasses-wearing nerd kid affectionately called chubby by my family. But if I were on Flag Team, life would be better, and maybe Justin would think I was cool. He had green eyes and sandy blonde hair and could play every sport.

So, I prepared for two weeks, holding straddle splits and front-to-back splits longer and longer each day. By the end of my prep, I still couldn't do splits, but I could do something incredible: hold my body still for excessive amounts of time. This skill of long-held stretching for epochs would eventually turn into a career before it backfired on me and revealed my body's true instabilities.

On the day of the audition, I had planned to run onto the gym floor doing a cartwheel into a round-off, followed by sliding into my best straddle-esque splits. After that, I'd jump up and chant a cheer for our school's team, the Falcons.

They announced my name. I positioned myself at the far edge of the gym away from the judges and then ran screaming toward them, "Go Falcons!" I started my cartwheel, and as my feet flew overhead, my heavy glasses shot off my face like a missile and slid across the floor with the hiss of an ice skater slicing through an infinite rink. I could hear where my glasses landed due to the collectively held breath in the gym, but I couldn't *see* where they were because I was so near-sighted. I remember crawling on hands and knees, patting the floor, feeling for them. Finally, one of the other hopefuls handed them to me, and I pushed through the cheer.

Sat down.

Didn't make Flag Girls. Didn't date Justin.

But I did turn that newfound stretch concentration I had into my lifeline.

Something in me woke up as I prepared for that audition. It pivoted my life toward yoga. I started checking out yoga books at the library, got a subscription to *Yoga Journal* magazine (this was 1984, after all), and found that stretching and splitting was actually something I *was* really good at. The yoga helped quell my anxiety and ultimately helped me face my eating disorder. Unfortunately, it also became a crutch for me. While I weaned myself off food issues, I birthed a new problem that my dad, the doctor, called "obsessive-compulsive stretching."

Years of practice and study passed, and I was *that girl* in the front of the class who could wrap both legs around her head and circle her clasped hands around her body like a limb jump rope. My yoga practice revealed to me that I was truly flexible. Even more than flexible, I was supremely mobile. I guess another way of saying this is: underneath my sedentary body was an underlying body type of hypermobility that would lead to chronic pain, degeneration, and surgeries all by the age of forty-five.

My yoga teachers and mentors encouraged me to teach because I could model poses just like them. What they didn't know in the 1980s and '90s is that they were about to close in on their own debilitating pain and degeneration issues because no one was truly practicing "safe yoga" for hypermobile students in this hall of mirrors.

In my early thirties, I became involved with the fascia research community in an attempt to help my own pain. Remarkably, I began to learn about the systemic issues that cluster with hypermobility. The one element that links hypermobility with a buffet of other surprising disorders is the foundational molecule within connective tissue—collagen. Fascia is loaded with collagen, and genetics frequently determine the natural tension and elasticity ranges within fascia. The bendy body types tend to proliferate laxity.

But collagen isn't just the foundational molecule within fascia and connective tissues. Collagen is the ubiquitous molecule that acts as a foundational substrate for every tissue in your body. When it's unruly, it can leave a bendy person feeling confused and betrayed by their own body. Research reveals that hypermobile bodies suffer from ongoing challenges from poor coordination, bizarre allergies, bowel problems, anxiety and eating disorders, fainting spells, early-onset arthritis, auto-immune complexity, cardiovascular issues, prolapse, vision problems (that explains my thick glasses at age twelve!), and so much more.

Being hypermobile makes it very difficult to sense where your own body begins and ends. It's much like doing cartwheels blind in a gymnasium where you can't see or feel the floor. For my first two decades of yoga practice in my teens and twenties, I roamed freely in the gaping joints and connective tissues of my body until it frayed at its edges. My next two decades were spent playing Whack-a-Mole with an ever-growing list of odd symptoms, chasing after what I now know as intertwined pathologies.

The past twenty years of my life have been successful in eliminating practices that were hastening my tissue's issues. It transformed my practice and career into one that educates others how to feel, see, hear, and understand what their body (whether hypermobile or not) is telling them and how to self-treat with self-myofascial release, body-mapping, and stability.

But my time did come. I had outlived a degenerating left hip that finally showed its disease to me after the birth of my second child. When my orthopedist assessed my forty-five-year-old painful hip at his clinic after viewing my bone-on-bone X-Ray, he circled my hip and said, "Well, there's your pre-existing condition right there—hypermobility."

I wonder if I had met Dr. Libby Hinsley in my twenties when I was really going for that end-range life, perhaps I could have learned to live in my body in a different way and still reap the benefits of yoga while managing my hypermobility. I'll never have that chance. But you, the reader, can and do have a new way of moving your practice in a healthy direction.

Libby has written a book that is both an intervention and a caution. I share my story as someone who has lived through the ravages of pushing a hypermobile body into unsafe body-based harm. At the time, I just didn't have the knowledge that I now have and teach to mitigate the march of time on a hypermobile body.

What you hold in your hands is a guidebook for yourself, your students, and even your offspring, who may carry genes

that veer toward hypermobility. This book will make a difference in your life. Read it, practice it, and trust this new road.

May your road to splits never land you in a splint. May your yoga journey be dynamic and stable, and may it bring you peace and joy. Above all, may it help you find you. I'll be waving a flag and cheering you on!

Jill Miller, C-IAYT, ERYT, author of *The Roll Model, Body by Breath*, and co-founder of Tune Up Fitness Worldwide

Book Introduction

———

I've always been good at party tricks.

From an early age, I could bend myself like a contortionist. This ability came in handy during childhood gymnastics classes and later in college yoga classes.

No stranger to extreme backbends and splits, I spent years flinging myself around my yoga mat in an impressively acrobatic way with a fervor only matched by all the other bendy yoga practitioners around me. When it came to my yoga practice, it was "go big or go home." Unfortunately, I ended up going home in pain on a regular basis.

I always knew I had generalized joint hypermobility, which is to say my joints move more than normal. What I didn't know until more recently, however, is that I have Hypermobile Ehlers-Danlos Syndrome (hEDS). I'll go into detail about hEDS later. For now, just know hEDS is a genetic connective tissue disorder that causes joint hypermobility and a variety of other challenges throughout the body—something I call being "bendy." Being bendy has truly shaped my life, in no way more profoundly than in my yoga experience.

The message I always received in yoga classes was to go deeper; stretch farther. So, I did, and I was praised for it. It was a nice ego boost when my less-bendy fellow students would say things like, "Wow, you're really good at yoga! Maybe someday I'll be able to do that too." But honestly, I remember being confused by the notion that being good at yoga was somehow linked to my bendy body.

What I didn't tell them was, "My body hurts all the time. I have chronic fatigue, a wide variety of food sensitivities, and sometimes debilitating anxiety and depression. I look healthy, but I'm suffering, and I'm not sure why."

I was the young, healthy-looking person getting MRIs on her knees because they hurt unexplainably, limping around at the end of the workday due to severe foot and hip pain, visiting chiropractor after chiropractor for help with my back and neck pain, and being way-laid by muscle spasms so severe I couldn't move my head for days.

Unfortunately, medical practitioners didn't notice my hypermobility, or if they did, they didn't recognize it was related to my various health issues. It simply wasn't on anyone's radar. Nothing ever seemed to be wrong with me, and imaging studies always came back normal.

I eventually turned more intensely to yoga and ultimately became a yoga instructor. I continued to do fast-paced, contortionist-style postures (usually in a heated room), inadvertently exploiting my hypermobility further. And I continued to be in pain.

In 2008, I traveled to Chennai, India, for a month-long yoga immersion at the Krishnamacharya Yoga Mandiram (KYM), a yoga center established by TKV Desikachar to pass on the teachings of his father Tirumalai Krishnamacharya, one of the most revered yoga masters of modern times (Krishnamacharya Yoga Mandiram 2019).

The experience was life-changing. It re-arranged everything I thought I knew about yoga and began to turn things around for my chronic injuries.

Full disclosure: I hated it at first.

The asana techniques were so different from what I had practiced before. I found the slow, mindful movement boring, and incredibly difficult! Slowing down revealed how challenging it was to control my movements without relying on momentum. As I'll discuss in this book, many bendy people share the same challenge.

I eventually came to learn this newfound approach to practice was exactly what I needed. It ultimately transformed my asana practice from a source of injury to one of healing. The breathing, meditation, and philosophical approach also brought a new richness to my practice, and I started to understand what yoga has to offer for personal transformation beyond asana.

Upon my return from India, I began training to be a physical therapist and eventually started my own physical therapy practice incorporating yoga as a primary treatment modality. Naturally, I ended up treating a lot of injured yoga practitioners.

I started noticing patterns among my yoga-practicing patients that were strikingly similar to my own life. Almost all of them had joint hypermobility contributing to their complaints and most practiced styles of asana that further exacerbated their problems. They all listed the same complaints I'd always struggled with, such as sacroiliac joint pain, hamstring strain, and shoulder pain, among others.

But that wasn't all. Many even shared similar struggles with mental health, digestive issues, pelvic floor dysfunction, and fatigue. Hypermobility was just the tip of the iceberg. I immersed myself in the literature on hypermobility and set about understanding how all these phenomena were interrelated.

Some estimate as much as 20 percent of the general population has joint hypermobility (Demmler et al. 2019). I suspect hypermobility is even more prevalent among yoga practitioners. If you're a yoga teacher, you likely see hypermobile students regularly. Bendy people are drawn to yoga for many reasons. Their natural ability to get into challenging yoga postures quickly propels them to *advanced* status. They may also have pain, anxiety, poor sleep, or other challenges that they hope yoga can alleviate.

Here's the catch: for many bendy practitioners, yoga isn't the balm they were hoping for. Instead, the practice further contributes to their pain and injuries. What's up with that? This book is my answer.

I've presented the book in three parts. Part One offers background information about yoga, hypermobility syndromes, and connective tissue. It also establishes a mindset for exploring the remainder of the book. In Part Two, I present key considerations for asana practice to support bendy people, including smaller and slower movements, stretching, strength and stability, and postural awareness. Part Two also offers recommendations for designing an asana practice and using verbal cues and hands-on assists wisely. Part Three considers how elements of yoga practice beyond asana, including self-massage, pranayama, relaxation, and meditation practices, can support people with hypermobility syndromes.

This book is for yoga teachers and therapists who want to understand hypermobility syndromes and develop a well-informed approach to yoga that fully supports bendy students without increasing their risk of injury. It's also for hypermobile practitioners seeking guidance on how to get the most benefit out of yoga practice.

I share this book to raise awareness and improve understanding of this important topic in the yoga community—and beyond. Yoga can be fabulous for people with hypermobility if practiced wisely. If practiced unwisely, it can be a recipe for chronic injury and pain. The devil is always in the details.

PART 1:

BACKGROUND

CHAPTER 1:

What is Yoga?

"The end goals of yoga are peace, freedom, contentment, and connection (union). A far cry from handstands and splits!"

Right out of the gate, we need to tackle the elephant that walks into the room anytime someone writes a book called *Yoga for...* (fill in the blank). While this book is about hypermobility, it's also about yoga, and there's a good deal of misunderstanding about both topics out there. Much of yoga's history and cultural significance has been lost in many modern Western yoga spaces. Many modern practitioners have lost sight of the ultimate goals of yoga, and this sets the stage for the challenges faced by bendy practitioners. Whether you're a yoga teacher or not, I hope you'll join me in reflecting on the question, "What is Yoga?"

Yoga is an ancient wisdom tradition developed over many hundreds of years in India. It has a complex history comprised of many branches and even divergent schools of thought (Feuerstein 1998).

Over the past few decades, yoga has become an increasingly popular practice in the West. The 2016 "Yoga in America" study by Yoga Alliance and *Yoga Journal* found 36 million people practice yoga in the US alone (Yoga Alliance 2021). As one of those practitioners, I am humbled to have the opportunity to learn and benefit from a wisdom tradition that is deeply entwined with a culture that is not my own. Holding onto threads of the yoga tradition in modern times is an important way to honor yoga's roots and avoid being swept up by the sterilized, stripped-down versions of yoga often presented in the media.

In the modern Western world, the physical practice of yoga postures called asanas has become synonymous with yoga. These days, it would be easy for a newcomer to assume yoga is about achieving challenging postures worthy of a magazine cover. But nothing could be further from the truth. Asana is just one component of the yoga tradition.

The word yoga comes from the Sanskrit root meaning "to join," indicating the practices and goals of yoga have something to do with connection or union (Feuerstein 1998). Although yoga has been described in various ways, it always points to an inner experience. In his thorough volume, *The Yoga Tradition* (1998), Georg Feuerstein opens his first chapter by stating:

> Yoga is a spectacularly multifaceted phenomenon...
> What all branches and schools of Yoga have in common,

however, is that they are concerned with a state of being, or consciousness, that is truly foundational.

This state of being is characterized by a deep understanding of one's true nature, connection to something greater than oneself, and ultimately, a sense of freedom from suffering (Desikachar 1999).

Although many yoga texts are worthy of mention, the *Yoga Sutras of Patanjali* is one of the most significant. Patanjali is the author credited with codifying what had previously been an oral tradition into a set of 195 sutras, or aphorisms, containing the wisdom of the yoga tradition (Desikachar 2008). Each sutra is to be interpreted and expounded upon by a master teacher. While the precise date of Patanjali's life and work is a topic of ongoing debate, the Yoga Sutras are estimated to be around 2,000 years old (Desikachar 2008).

The second sutra defines yoga as "the ability to direct the mind exclusively toward an object and sustain that direction without any distraction" (Desikachar 1999). In other words, yoga is about taming the mind's wild ups and downs to achieve a state of inner calm.

But yoga wants us to focus the mind for a specific reason. The third sutra goes on to say, "Then, the ability to understand the object fully and correctly is apparent" (Desikachar 2008). The object of our attention and study in yoga is ourselves. When we understand who we are, our actions are more likely to decrease suffering for ourselves and others.

Kristine Kaoverii Weber, yoga teacher and founder of Subtle Yoga, described it elegantly in a recent conversation we had:

> The practices of yoga can lead you to a deeper sense of who you are, and to a sense of meaning and purpose. When you know who you are, you know how to be in the world. You know what to do with yourself. And that's really the goal of yoga—to get to know yourself better, understand yourself better, and develop a better relationship with yourself so you can be present with yourself and the world—and offer the best of yourself in the spirit of service.

In a sense, yoga is about paying attention, and the tools of yoga help us learn and practice this undervalued skill. Paying attention is the key to freeing ourselves from unexamined (and sometimes destructive) habits that keep us stuck in a cycle of suffering. In *The Heart of Yoga* (1999), T.K.V. Desikachar states:

> Yoga attempts to create a state in which we are always present—really present—in every action, in every moment. The advantage of attentiveness is that we perform each task better and, at the same time, are conscious of our actions.... When we are attentive to our actions, we are not prisoners to our habits....

In *The Yoga Sutras*, Patanjali outlines an eight-limbed path to understand and optimize the mind, decrease suffering, and reach our highest potential as human beings. The eight limbs of yoga are as follows: yama, niyama, asana, pranayama, pratyahara, dharana, dhyana, and samadhi (Desikachar 2008).

The first two limbs of yoga—yama and niyama—offer an ethical framework for life. Essentially, they're about paying attention to our behavior. They provide an outline for how to be nice to others (yamas) and how to be nice to ourselves (niyamas). The yamas include ahimsa, or non-violence; satya, or truthfulness; asteya, or non-stealing; brahmacarya, or moderation; and aparigraha, or non-hoarding. The niyamas include sauca, or cleanliness; samtosha, or contentment; tapas, or inner effort; svadhyaya, or self-study; and isvara-pranidhana, or surrender to the Divine.

The third limb of yoga is asana, the practice of physical postures. Next comes pranayama, the breath practices designed to nourish and balance the subtle energy called "prana." Pratyahara is the withdrawal of the senses to guide our attention more deeply inward. Dharana is the process of intense concentration, and dhyana is the process of understanding through meditation. Finally, samadhi is the practice of absorption (or union).

I like the way Tim Gard et al. (2014) describe the eight limbs of yoga as essentially presenting four main tools for promoting self-regulation. They define self-regulation broadly: "...*self-regulation* refers to efforts of monitoring, willpower, and motivation to manage or alter one's incipient responses and impulses so as to pursue or maintain explicit goals or standards."

In other words, self-regulation is the ability to decrease our moment-to-moment emotional reactivity that so often leads to behaviors that increase our (and others') suffering. Self-regulation helps us gain perspective and a deeper understanding of ourselves. In that state, it's easier to make better decisions and behave in ways that align with our values.

The four key domains they describe are ethics (limbs 1 and 2), postures (limb 3), breathing (limb 4), and meditative practices (limbs 5–8).

Each step along the eight limbs takes us further into the interior of our experience along a path of progressive subtlety. The end goals of yoga are peace, freedom, contentment, and connection (union). A far cry from handstands and splits!

Asana is the entry point for most yoga practitioners, and there's nothing wrong with that. A mindful asana practice can help us learn about and take care of our bodies. It can help us fully arrive in the present moment and learn to pay attention to our experience as it happens. Within asana practice, we can study our habits, our breath, our thoughts, and our emotions.

In the larger context of yoga, asana is not an end in and of itself but rather a tool to help us develop the self-understanding and self-regulation that can lead to better choices about how we live. Does asana have to be fancy to accomplish this? No, it doesn't. *Can* it be fancy to accomplish this? Sure. But simple asana and fancy asana are equal in their ability to guide us inward for the purpose of yoga.

When we reduce yoga to the performance of asanas for their own sake, we miss out on the other tools of yoga and strip asana of its broader function within the context of yoga. Asana *as performance* is also what leads to injury, especially for bendy yoga practitioners. That's because the yoga asana aesthetic glorifies hypermobility as an asset rather than the liability it often is.

I was recently lucky enough to have a conversation with Judith Hanson Lasater, a yoga teacher for more than fifty years and a physical therapist who holds a PhD in East-West Psychology. In our conversation, she reflected on a common misunderstanding of the word asana.

> The practice of yoga is a big umbrella and includes philosophy, asana practice, breathing, and meditation. Asana is a part of it, but many people in our culture conflate the practice of asana with the whole of yoga, and many even narrow it down more and interpret the word yoga as the practice of asana in a hot environment. But when I say "yoga practice," I specifically mean a broad umbrella. And when I say "asana," I simply and only mean the practice of asana.

In my years of training yoga teachers, I have observed a reluctance to let go of the over-identification with asana performance. Despite having been touched by the inner experience of yoga practice, they tend to gravitate toward performative asana and the never-ending quest for more mobility. It's a habit that is exquisitely difficult to break. I have great compassion for it because that used to be me.

Soon after I returned from studying at the Krishnamacharya Yoga Mandiram (KYM) in Chennai, India, I attended a yoga workshop in Chapel Hill, North Carolina, with a revered yoga teacher who was trained in the same lineage.

While my practice had begun to change because of my experience at the KYM, you could still find me flinging myself around my mat at the power vinyasa class, enjoying the momentum and the heat. I had one foot in two different yoga worlds. My old way of practicing was perpetuating a cycle of chronic pain and injury.

I was toward the end of my ten-year run with a chronic hamstring strain (pain where the hamstring muscles attach to the sitting bone) and sacroiliac joint pain. I was excited to ask this yoga teacher about my troubles. When I had my moment during lunch one day, I swallowed my nervousness and approached him with my heart racing. I said, "Can I ask you about my chronic hamstring strain? I've had it for many years, and I just can't seem to get rid of it."

As if he'd heard this question a thousand times from young vinyasa fanatics (he probably had), he made a hint of an eye roll and said, "You have to stop forward folding." He said a few other clarifying words, but all I could hear was, "*You have to stop forward folding,*" as it echoed around inside my head.

Stop forward folding? Was he insane? If you'd looked at my practice at that time, you'd think I believed enlightenment lived in the hamstrings. Deep forward folds were the name of the game. To stop seemed unthinkable.

On my drive home from Chapel Hill at the end of the weekend, I was mulling over this teacher's recommendation about forward folding, thinking about the unthinkable. I realized how identified I had become with my ability to perform impressive postures, and I knew I had a decision to make.

Was I going to continue the popular styles of asana that weren't working for me? Or was I going to embrace the new ways of practicing I had discovered at the KYM? I chose the latter, and I even decided to try his recommendation about forward folding. It wasn't without some trepidation. What would people think when I skipped the forward folds in class? Would they judge me as a bad yoga practitioner or teacher?

When I attended asana classes, I substituted chair pose for all the standing forward folds, and I got creative with other posture modifications too. My trepidation faded, and I came to enjoy my newfound freedom. I felt empowered to take charge of my body and make my own decisions about asana practice. The other good news: after about a year of these modifications, my chronic hamstring strain finally healed and hasn't bothered me since.

When I make similar suggestions to my hypermobile students and patients with the same chronic complaints I used to have, they make the same face I must have made in 2009 when that teacher suggested I drop the forward folds. I imagine my words echoing around in their minds as they wonder how I got to be crazy enough to suggest the unthinkable.

It may not be about forward folds, but my guidance is always the same: Be willing to change your practice so that it serves your needs instead of contributing to your pain and suffering. That usually means dropping your identification with aesthetics and performance.

Somewhere along the way, the ability to perform difficult stretchy yoga postures became confused with "advanced yoga." Media representations of yoga often depict a lithe person in an aesthetically impressive posture that appears impossible for the run-of-the-mill human to achieve (because it is). As I mentioned before, the conflation of yoga with asana performance has much to do with the challenges facing hypermobile practitioners.

The over-emphasis on performance leads hypermobile practitioners to exploit their mobility at the risk of injury. It also intimidates many other would-be practitioners and likely prevents them from beginning a practice that could positively impact their lives. People who can contort themselves into challenging positions are encouraged and praised for being good at yoga, while those who can't do such things end up thinking they are *not good* at yoga.

For example, people who require a chair for yoga practice due to difficulty getting to the floor may mistakenly believe they are doing remedial yoga, and if they're lucky, one day they'll graduate to *real* yoga.

I frequently ask my yoga teacher trainees to repeat aloud after me: *"There is no remedial yoga."* Even though they chuckle for a moment, a visible change comes over their faces. It's a look of relief, not only for their future students but also for themselves. Compassion emerges for how they've judged themselves, their physical abilities, and their limitations.

No matter what some media representations of yoga might have you believe, advanced yoga has nothing to do with difficult postures. Yoga isn't interested in how your yoga postures look or how bendy your body is. Nailing a split doesn't help you attain the goals of yoga any more quickly or any more truly. I wish it were that easy.

The common confusion between asana performance and "advanced yoga" reminds me of a Zen koan (like a riddle) I learned many years ago: "Don't mistake your finger for the moon."

In the context of yoga, we could say the moon represents the state of being that is yoga—one of self-understanding, peace, and connection. The finger represents the tools and practices of yoga designed to point us toward that state of being. If we aren't careful, we may conflate the finger that points to the moon with the moon itself and get caught up with the performance of a particular asana as though it is the end goal.

In his book, *Old Path White Clouds: Walking in the Footsteps of the Buddha*, the revered Buddhist monk and teacher Thich Nhat Hanh described it this way:

> Bhikkhus, the teaching is merely a vehicle to describe the truth. Don't mistake it for the truth itself. A finger pointing at the moon is not the moon. The finger is needed to know where to look for the moon, but if you mistake the finger for the moon itself, you will never know the real moon. The teaching is like a raft that carries you to the other shore. The raft is needed, but the raft is not the other shore. An intelligent person would not carry the raft around on his head after making it across to the other shore....

The goal isn't to achieve certain postures and carry them around like trophies, and certainly not at the risk of our own pain and injury. Ultimately, yoga is about feeling good! Not just a fleeting momentary good, but a deep abiding good that comes from understanding who you are, knowing your connection to others, and aligning your actions with your highest values. The details of outward appearance are far less relevant than the inner experience of the practitioner.

Now that we've got our bearings on some yoga basics, I'm going to take you on a deep dive into the world of joint hyper-mobility syndromes in the remainder of Part One. Then, we will explore yoga for bendy people—not just asana for bendy people, but all of it.

CHAPTER 2:

Hypermobility 101

———

"Sometimes when you hear hoofbeats, it really is a zebra."

—THE EHLERS-DANLOS SOCIETY (2021)

Since this is a book about yoga for bendy people, let's take a moment to clarify what it means to be bendy. The term "hypermobility" describes a joint's ability to move beyond the normal range of motion. So, let's start there.

Range of motion describes how far a joint can move in any given direction. For every joint in the body, "normal" or typical ranges of motion have been established based on what researchers observe in human beings. Although human bodies are variable, most people's joint range of motion falls somewhere in the vicinity of "normal" (barring injury or surgery).

Let's explore shoulder flexion, which is taking the arm forward and up. Normal shoulder flexion range of motion is 180 degrees, with the arm straight overhead beside the ear. If I take my arm out in front of me just a little bit to open my car door, I'm using my shoulder in "mid-range" flexion. If I take my arm up in front of me all the way, such as to hang from a jungle gym at 180 degrees, I'm using my shoulder at "end-range" flexion.

Range of motion can be achieved actively or passively. Active shoulder flexion is when I use the strength of my own arm muscles to lift it up as far as it will go. Passive shoulder flexion occurs when someone (or something) else lifts it up for me (Magee 2008). It's common for joints to demonstrate greater passive range of motion versus active range of motion.

Let's consider hip external rotation. If I lie on my back and bend my right knee so my knee is over my hip and my shin is parallel to the floor, I can observe the difference between active and passive right hip external rotation range of motion.

When I use my leg muscles to actively rotate my hip externally as far as I can, it goes a little more than 45 degrees such that my knee cap points diagonally out to the right (See Figure 2a). The limit of active range of motion is sometimes referred to as the physiological barrier (Magee 2008).

But if I cross my right ankle over my left knee and bring my left knee toward my chest, the movement of my left knee will push my right hip farther into external rotation passively. Then my right knee points 90 degrees to the right (See Figure 2b). This passive external rotation limit is known as the anatomical barrier (Magee 2008).

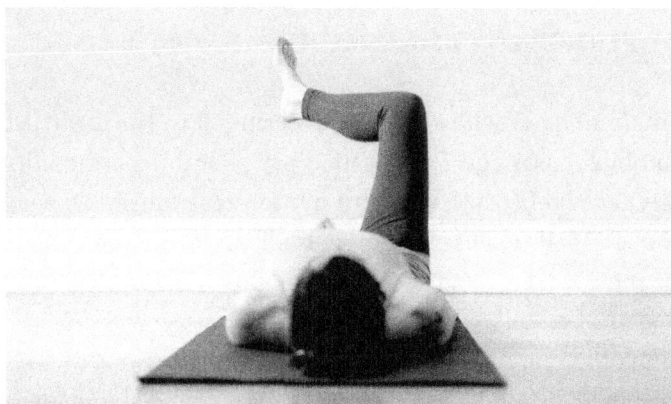

Figure 2a

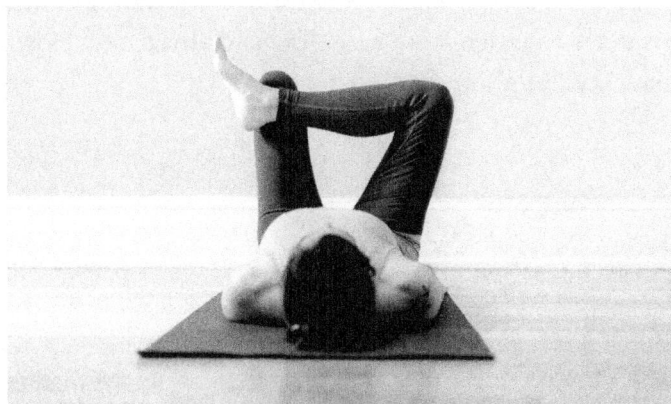

Figure 2b

Normal range of motion for hip external rotation is between 40–60 degrees (Magee 2008). What I'm demonstrating here is an example of hypermobility.

HYPERMOBILITY ASSESSMENT

There are several types of joint hypermobility. Having hyper-mobile hands and feet is called peripheral hypermobility. Hypermobility in fewer than five joints is called localized hypermobility, whereas hypermobility in five or more joints is considered generalized hypermobility (Castori et al. 2017).

The most commonly used hypermobility assessment tool is the Beighton Scale. It assesses standing forward fold, knee and elbow hyperextension, and thumb and pinky finger hypermobility for a total possible score of nine (See Figures 2c-2g). A score of four or more (or five, depending on the study) is considered indicative of generalized joint hyper-mobility (Bockhorn et al. 2021).

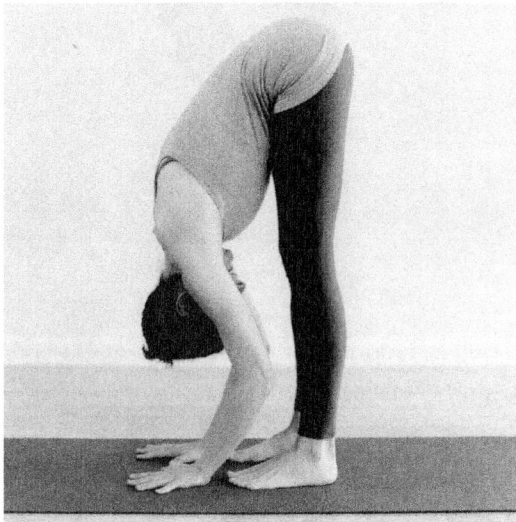

Figure 2c

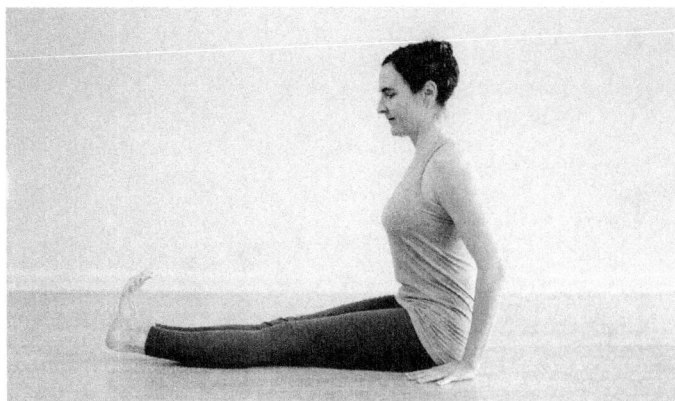

Figure 2d

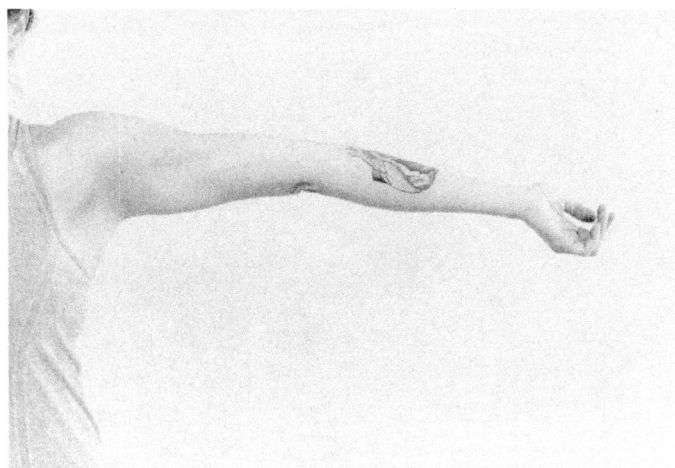

Figure 2e

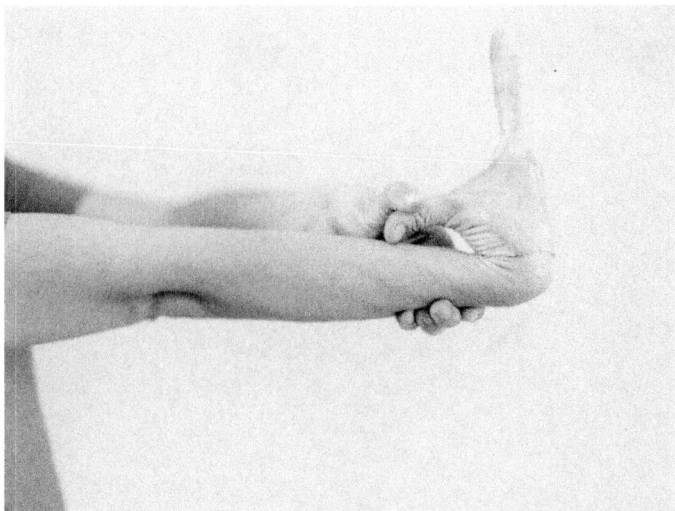

Figure 2f

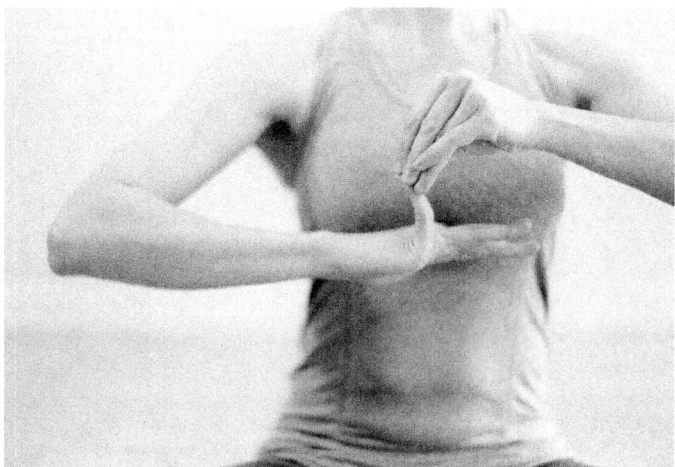

Figure 2g

Since the Beighton Scale assesses so few joints in the body, other measures can help obtain a more comprehensive assessment of hypermobility. These include the Lower Limb Assessment Score (Meyer 2017) and the Upper Limb Assessment Tool (Nicholson 2018). These tools examine the upper and lower extremities in more detail and can be useful, particularly for people with suspected generalized hypermobility but low Beighton scores.

Importantly, since most bodies become stiffer with age, a person's score on any of these assessment tools is likely to change over time. Hence, when assessing joint hypermobility, a person's history is relevant.

The five-point questionnaire on hypermobility (5PQ) is another tool used to assess hypermobility which specifically takes a person's history into account. It grants a point for each of the five questions, even if the person can't currently perform the task but could when they were younger. For example, it asks whether a person can, or ever could, touch their thumb to their forearm, and so on. A score of two or higher is indicative of generalized hypermobility (Glans et al. 2020).

In the most basic terms, joint hypermobility is just a description. It's neither a diagnosis nor an indication of pathology in and of itself. Several factors determine a joint's range of motion, including bone shape, muscle tension, and the laxity of the ligaments, tendons, and joint capsule surrounding it. So, just because someone scores high on the Beighton

Scale, for example, doesn't necessarily mean there's a problem. Some people have joint hypermobility without any symptoms.

Similarly, just because someone scores below a four on the Beighton Scale doesn't mean they *don't* have joint hypermobility. It seems counter-intuitive, but a hypermobile person's excessive joint range of motion isn't always obvious at first glance. That's because joint mobility isn't the same as flexibility.

MOBILITY VS. FLEXIBILITY

People often use "mobility" and "flexibility" interchangeably, but these terms describe different things. For our purposes, mobility is the movement available to a joint due to bone shape and the joint capsule and ligaments surrounding it. Flexibility is the movement available to a joint due to muscle strength, length, and resting tone (tension in the muscle at rest).

Dr. Linda Bluestein is a former ballet dancer, integrative medicine physician, and board-certified anesthesiologist who specializes in treating people with hypermobility syndromes. In a recent conversation I had with her, she described it like this:

> One of the biggest confusions is the difference between hypermobility and flexibility. Hypermobility has to do with what's going on in the bones, the ligaments which connect bone to bone, and the tendons which

connect muscle to bone…. Hypermobility refers specifically to what's going on in the joint, whereas flexibility refers more to the ability of the muscle and nervous system to use the range of motion that the joints have…. When people have joint hypermobility, they can actually end up with really tight muscles because the muscles are struggling to try to get some stabilization inside of the joint.

Increased mobility doesn't always correlate with increased muscle flexibility. As Dr. Bluestein described, many people with hypermobility struggle with muscle tension. In the following chapters, I'll explain more about this and other common bendy body complaints.

HYPERMOBILITY SYNDROMES

I mentioned above that a variety of factors determine how much a joint is able to move, including bone shape, muscle tension, and connective tissue laxity. In many cases, hypermobility is caused by an underlying genetic difference in the collagen (or the cells that produce collagen) within connective tissue (Malek and Koster 2021).

These genetic differences lead to more laxity (or floppiness, as I like to call it) in connective tissues that contain collagen, such as joint capsules, ligaments, tendons, and fascia. The result is joint hypermobility that is more likely to be associated with increased injury risk (Magee 2008) and symptoms across multiple systems of the body (Atwell et al. 2021). That's when it's referred to as a joint hypermobility syndrome or disorder.

Many genetic connective tissue disorders include hypermobility as a prominent feature, including Marfan Syndrome, Loeys-Dietz Syndrome, Osteogenesis Imperfecta, and the Ehlers-Danlos Syndromes. The most common of these are the Ehlers-Danlos Syndromes (EDS). There are currently fourteen identified subtypes of EDS, most of which are considered rare or ultra-rare diseases (EDS Types 2021).

Overall, EDS is characterized by joint hypermobility, skin hyperextensibility (extra stretchy skin), and tissue fragility (slow healing and impaired scarring) (Parapia and Jackson 2008). Chronic pain is also highly prevalent among people with EDS (Voermans et al. 2010). All subtypes result from a genetic defect in collagen or other components of connective tissue. However, there are many types of collagen, and many genes are involved in its production, assembly, and function. As the Ehlers-Danlos Society states on its website:

> There are many proteins in connective tissue. One of the key proteins is collagen. In the Ehlers-Danlos syndromes, there are faults in the genes that determine how the body makes collagen or, in some subtypes, other proteins that work alongside collagen. This leads to the connective tissue becoming weaker. Different tissues and organs can be affected in diverse ways depending on the genetic fault. This explains why there are several subtypes of EDS (What are the Ehlers-Danlos Syndromes 2021).

The overall combined prevalence of the Ehlers-Danlos Syndromes is between 1 in 3,500 to 1 in 5,000 people (What are the Ehlers-Danlos Syndromes 2021). However, most subtypes are rare, meaning they affect one in 40,000–200,000 people, and some are ultra-rare, meaning they affect fewer than one in a million people. The rarer forms of EDS include Vascular EDS and Classical EDS, among others, and some are associated with more severe disabilities.

For example, Vascular EDS (vEDS) is characterized by a gene mutation that most often affects Type III collagen, leading to fragile arteries and internal organs. People with vEDS are at risk for serious and life-threatening complications, including spontaneous colon rupture or arterial rupture (Byers et al. 2017). Classical EDS (cEDS) is characterized by a different genetic mutation affecting Type V collagen and leads to skin fragility, easy bruising, and impaired scarring, in addition to generalized joint hypermobility (Bowen et al. 2017).

HYPERMOBILE EDS AND HYPERMOBILITY SPECTRUM DISORDER

Of all the subtypes, the Hypermobile type (hEDS) is the most common. However, it remains the only one without a clear genetic marker. All other EDS subtypes can be diagnosed via a blood test.

While clarity about the specific genetic cause of hEDS has been elusive (Malek and Koster 2021), a couple of extensive research studies that hope to identify the genetic variation(s) underlying it are underway. Some recent research suggests hEDS may be caused by the impaired functionality of the cells that produce collagen (Malek and Koster 2021). Others suggest it may be associated with altered genes that regulate systemic inflammation (Makol et al. 2021).

In 2017, the International Consortium on EDS and related disorders updated and clarified all the Ehlers-Danlos Syndromes' diagnostic criteria, in part to support ongoing genetic research. Their work narrowed down the diagnostic criteria for Hypermobile EDS, which decreased the number of people who qualify for the diagnosis.

The hEDS diagnostic criteria include a person's score on the Beighton Scale and much more. Other elements include dental history, presence of abdominal hernias, chronic musculoskeletal pain, wingspan to height ratio (distance from fingertip to fingertip compared to height), and others (hEDS Diagnostic Checklist 2021). Many people have symptoms similar to that of hEDS but do not meet the diagnostic criteria. Those people are given the newly-developed diagnosis of Hypermobility Spectrum Disorder (HSD) (What are the Ehlers-Danlos Syndromes 2021).

Practically speaking, this means we now have two diagnoses for people with similar and overlapping symptoms.

Hypermobile EDS (hEDS) is diagnosed when specific criteria are met and when other connective tissue disorders are ruled out. Hypermobility Spectrum Disorder (HSD) is diagnosed when someone does not meet all the hEDS criteria but has hypermobility with associated symptoms, and other connective tissue disorders have been ruled out. If this seems confusing, join the club!

Many people mistakenly believe HSD is a lesser diagnosis than hEDS. However, people with HSD can have the same or greater severity of symptoms. This is not only misunderstood by patients but also by medical practitioners who aren't well-educated about the nuances of these conditions. As Dr. Bluestein explained in our recent talk:

> You can have hypermobility spectrum disorders that have just as much pain and just as much disability. You can still have all the same comorbidities, but a lot of people feel that the EDS diagnosis…carries more weight within the healthcare field.

Medical experts who treat hypermobility syndromes increasingly lump HSD/hEDS together due to their clinical similarities (Aubry-Rozier et al. 2021). Since they are essentially interchangeable for practical purposes, you'll often see HSD/hEDS discussed as one umbrella concept. That's how I will refer to it from here on out.

When I say HSD/hEDS, I'm talking about the broad category of people with symptomatic hypermobility when all other heritable connective tissue disorders have been ruled out. This is also what I mean by "bendy" moving forward. How many people are bendy? The prevalence of HSD/hEDS is difficult to estimate because it is so often misdiagnosed or missed altogether. But a recent study in Wales found a combined prevalence of HSD/hEDS to be 1 in 500, suggesting HSD/hEDS is not rare at all (Demmler et al. 2019).

MEDICAL KNOWLEDGE GAP

If you've wondered why zebra imagery pops up when you search for information about hypermobility, it's because the zebra has become a mascot of sorts for HSD/EDS. Medical providers are taught, "When you hear hoofbeats behind you, don't expect to see a zebra." In other words, they are trained to expect an ordinary diagnosis rather than a more surprising or less-common one. Many providers still consider HSD/hEDS a rare condition. Consequently, very few have a solid understanding of it.

HSD and hEDS are complex conditions and, unfortunately, are not well understood. They don't fit well within a singular medical specialty, making them difficult to diagnose and treat. If you peruse the literature on hypermobility, you'll find research from various disciplines, including rheumatology, orthopedics, and even psychiatry.

Dr. Andrew Beaumont is a neurosurgeon and yoga therapist in Wisconsin with an interest in hypermobility syndromes. During a recent conversation with him, we discussed the gap in knowledge about hypermobility syndromes among the medical community and how it negatively impacts patient care. He described one of the underlying causes for this:

> One of the problems is that in modern medicine, HSD and EDS are in a no man's land of interest because they touch on so many specialties. Patients are sent to a variety of specialists to address symptoms, but there's not one specialty that really owns the condition.

Due to the lack of understanding about these conditions, many patients struggle for years to understand their symptoms and receive a diagnosis that validates their experience and leads to effective treatment. Many people with hypermobility syndromes don't manifest symptoms the way medical doctors are trained to expect. As a result, they are often met with responses such as, "But you look so healthy," "You're too young to have all these problems," or "You can't have that; it's too rare." I was one of those patients.

The dismissal, denial, or trivialization of a patient's concerns by their doctor or other healthcare provider is called "medical gaslighting," and it can have damaging effects (Davis 2020). It delays or prevents patients from receiving a proper diagnosis and treatment for their condition. It can also cause patients to doubt their own experience and feel alone in their struggle for adequate care.

Unfortunately, when we don't understand our symptoms and don't receive any reassurance, validation, or clarity from our medical providers, fear often takes over. During my recent interview with Dr. Beaumont, we talked about how fear can make symptoms even worse.

> As a species, we're so fearful when we get a symptom and we don't know what it is. I'm the same way. You start panicking, and then that fuels the autonomic nervous system to be more activated, and then the pain is more severe. It's a vicious cycle.

Sometimes, diagnosis can be seen as a label that limits us. On the other hand, it can also help us make sense of our experience. Once we understand what's happening in our body, symptoms become less scary. They may not become less severe right away but turning down the fear makes it easier to actively engage in the process of healing. Dr. Beaumont described the change he sees in many of his patients after they receive an official diagnosis.

I've seen so many patients go through a transformation when they find a diagnosis and suddenly start to make sense of their symptoms. They come back and see me, and they're different people as they go through this journey of exploring and understanding. Their symptoms aren't necessarily better at the beginning, but emotionally and psychologically, they've made a huge leap. And the rest can follow after that.

My sincere hope is that people with undiagnosed hypermobility syndromes find the resources they need to validate their experience, understand their symptoms, and engage meaningfully in the process of healing. Although I'm focusing on HSD/hEDS in this book, I want to acknowledge again the variety of other forms of EDS and other inherited connective tissue disorders that also include joint hypermobility. Each of them deserves equally focused attention. If any suggestions in this book are helpful for people who have those conditions, I will be very glad about that.

If you're a yoga teacher, it's likely you see people with joint hypermobility on a regular basis. You may notice people getting into contortionist types of postures with ease, dropping into a split like it's no big deal, or clasping hands easily behind them in the cow's face pose (See Figure 2h).

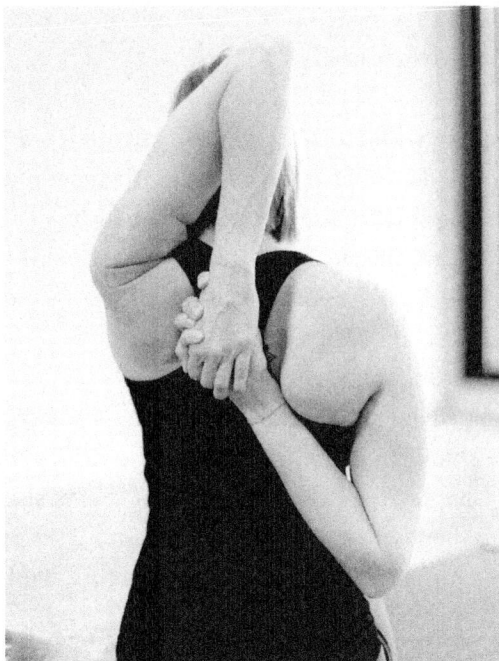

Figure 2h

Keep in mind there's a giant leap between observing someone's impressive mobility in your class and diagnosing them
with a hypermobility syndrome. However, yoga teachers are
in a unique position to raise awareness about hypermobility,
have conversations, and ask questions that may lead someone
to a greater understanding of their condition.

If you're a yoga teacher and a student reports symptoms
they or you think are related to hypermobility, an in-depth
examination is warranted. A good place to start is with their
primary care physician or physical therapist. If someone's
concerns aren't validated by their medical provider, I always

recommend they switch providers until they find someone responsive to their needs.

Many people with HSD/hEDS do best with a team of supportive providers to help them manage their symptoms and co-occurring conditions. That team often includes a primary care physician, physical therapist, mental health provider, and specialists as needed from gastroenterology, cardiology, rheumatology, and others.

In the next chapter, I'll explore the nitty-gritty of connective tissue to elucidate the basis for hypermobility syndromes. Then in Chapter 4, I'll describe some of the most common challenges bendy people face to paint a more thorough picture of what it means to have a hypermobility syndrome.

After a lifetime of oddities and injuries, things fell apart after the birth of my second child in 2016, two months shy of my fortieth birthday. It started with some heel pain that came out of the blue and eventually progressed to severe pain in both feet that prevented me from walking barefoot for about eighteen months. Over and over again, I would report to people, "It feels like I don't have fat pads on my feet. I just can't stand the pressure!"

I'll never forget having to get a pristine clean pair of special sneakers designed to relieve heel pain (they were magic) to wear at the yoga studio where I taught and attended classes. I squeaked around the studio, often joking I was trying to set a new yoga trend.

One day, I was attending a yoga class in my sneakers, and as everyone was settling in for class, another student rushed over to me, trying to catch me before I defiled another inch of the sacred yoga studio floor. With a scornful face, she barked at me, "Don't you know, you can't wear shoes in here!"

This was a woman I had seen many times around the studio where I had taught for sixteen years, and her remark took me off guard. I initially thought she was joking, but the prolonged and unchanging look on her face told me otherwise.

I stammered, "Oh, I have a problem with my feet, and I have to wear shoes.... These shoes are clean...I only wear them here...I work here..." My words trailed off as I retreated slowly to my mat, still confused, a little embarrassed, and more self-conscious about my situation.

Much later, I learned the fat pads on the bottom of the feet can herniate through the superficial fascia, creating little visible pockets of tissue that stick out the sides of the heels when you're standing. They're called piezogenic papules, and they are one of the signs of hEDS. When I learned about this, I stood up, examined my feet, and lo and behold! I have those. No wonder it felt as though I didn't have fat pads.

During that time, I also developed widespread joint pain, fatigue, heart palpitations, brain fog bad enough to get me lost a few times in the same neighborhood where I had lived for fifteen years, and deepening depression.

I saw four physical therapists, two acupuncturists, two naturopaths, and an integrative MD. I had piles and piles of lab work done. Aside from a couple of fine-tuning things here and there, nothing could ever explain my symptoms. Every time something appeared that seemed even on the edge of normal, I jumped on it with renewed hope that maybe *this was it*.

I eventually went to see a handful of specialists. The rheumatologist, gastroenterologist, and cardiologist were all equally at a loss for how to help me. While each of those experiences is story-worthy, the cardiologist takes the cake.

I went there due to near-constant heart palpitations and inability to walk up my stairs without feeling like I'd just run a marathon. My fatigue was indescribable. I thought I must be dying. In yoga class, I couldn't hold my arms up overhead without getting dizzy and feeling like my heart would jump out of my chest. At the end of my visit with the cardiologist, he said, "Whelp, there's almost no chance there's anything wrong with you." Shocked, I said, "You mean, after never having heart palpitations in my life, you're telling me it's normal to have them all day, every day?" To which he replied, "Yes."

Unfortunately, he never considered that I might have POTS (Postural Orthostatic Tachycardia Syndrome), and at that point, I'd never heard of it either. POTS is one of the most common comorbidities (co-occurring conditions) among people with HSD/hEDS. It occurs when a person's heart rate elevates beyond normal amounts upon coming to an upright position (Cleveland Clinic 2021). Some months later, I learned how to test myself for POTS...ding ding ding!

I continued my own research and began suspecting I might have hEDS. I always knew I had joint hypermobility. In the context of my clinical work with patients who have hypermobility and chronic pain, I started connecting some dots. I downloaded the diagnostic criteria for hEDS. From what I could tell, it was a match. When I presented it to my primary care doctor, she sent me to the medical geneticist for confirmation.

My visit with the geneticist was my first telehealth experience at the beginning of the COVID-19 pandemic. As he appeared on the screen, I immediately searched his office for signs of hope. I saw a picture of his family in his office and the usual stacks of books and medical journals surrounding him. He seemed about my age, wore comfortingly thick-rimmed glasses, and his voice was kind. I thought, "Okay, he cares about his family, he reads a lot, he looks relatable.... So far, so good."

In sharp contrast to the length of time it took me to finally end up at this telehealth visit, his evaluation was brief. I described my symptoms and my life to him as I had done so many times before. But he didn't respond as everyone else had. He didn't look at me with confusion, irritation, or a dismissive eye roll. He didn't try to tell me there was nothing wrong with me. His face showed familiarity and understanding. He said,

> I have some questions to ask you, and I'll have you show me a few things, but I can tell you just from talking with you and reading over your paperwork, this sounds like a classic case of Hypermobile EDS.

The relief and validation I felt at that moment was unspeakable. Recalling it still brings a lump to my throat. As the Ehlers-Danlos Society says on its website, "Sometimes when you hear hoofbeats, it really is a zebra" (Why the Zebra 2021).

Suddenly, my life made sense, and I knew I wasn't crazy. The reason my body never seemed to be quite like my peers was because it wasn't. I have a different body. My diagnosis gave me the permission to finally listen to my different body and learn how to take care of it. As strange as it may sound, it set me free.

CHAPTER 3:

Connective Tissue Nitty-Gritty

"Like a rubber band, elastin is able to stretch and then return right back to its original length. Collagen is nothing like a rubber band; it's like a steel cable."

In the previous chapter, I discussed how hypermobility syndromes are the result of genetic differences that impact the structure and function of connective tissue. This chapter is heavy on the technical and science-y stuff. It's meant for those who want to dive deeper into what connective tissue is all about.

CONNECTIVE TISSUE

Connective tissue has become quite a buzzword in recent years. I've been in more than a few yoga classes in which the teacher touts the benefits of the practice for my connective tissue, so let's clarify some terms.

Connective tissue is a broad umbrella term that includes tendons, ligaments, joint capsules, fascia, and bone, as well as adipose tissue (fat) and blood. In general, connective tissues connect, support, and bind together other tissues and perform myriad functions all on their own (Stecco 2015; Kamrami et al. 2021). I'm going to focus on ligaments, tendons, joint capsules, and fascia—tissues made largely of collagen.

These tissues are comprised of structural proteins of varying densities, including collagen and elastin, fibroblast cells (which produce collagen, among other things), and other components. All of those components are surrounded by viscous (thick and gluey) fluid called the extracellular matrix (Stecco 2015; Kamrami et al. 2021).

Collagen and elastin are the most common structural proteins in connective tissue, although collagen is far more abundant. In fact, collagen is the most abundant protein in your body (Kendall and Feghall-Bostwick 2014).

Like a rubber band, elastin is able to stretch and then return right back to its original length. Collagen is nothing like a rubber band; it's like a steel cable. Its superpower is resisting tensile force, otherwise known as stretching (Stecco 2015). Collagen-rich tissues have some give to them, but not much.

That's a good thing, since collagen is basically the glue that holds your body together.

There are over twenty-five different types of collagen in the body and somewhere around forty different genes involved in its production, assembly, and function (Arseni et al. 2018).

FASCIA

Fascia is one type of collagenous connective tissue that surrounds, separates, and binds together muscles, organs, and other tissues. Most agree there are several kinds of fascia (Kumka and Bonar 2012). Many describe them as superficial, deep or investing, and visceral (Stecco 2015). Even though these terms aren't perfect, they'll be adequate for our purposes.

Superficial fascia lies underneath your skin, keeping your skin attached to your body. Deep (sometimes called investing) fascia consists of thicker sheaths of tissue that separate muscle compartments and form sturdier structures, such as the thick thoracolumbar fascia in your lower back (Willard 2012). Visceral fascia surrounds organs, nerves, and vessels and allows all the tissues of the body to slide and glide along each other, making way for easeful movement.

You may have heard the term "myofascia" in various yoga and movement settings. "Myo" refers to muscle, and "fascia" refers to collagen-rich fascia. Muscle is never separate from fascia, although fascia is sometimes separate from muscle. When they're together, they make up the myofascial system.

Each muscle has a beginning and an end; we call these its "attachment sites." Fascia has no beginning or end; it's continuous throughout the body (Stecco 2015).

Fascia that is integrated into muscle tissue is referred to as myofascia. Every muscle cell is surrounded by and connected to its neighboring cells by a thin layer of fascia. Muscle fibers are grouped together to form fascicles which are also surrounded by a layer of fascia. Many muscle fascicles are then grouped together to form a muscle unit that is surrounded by yet another fascial layer (Purslow and Delage 2012). Myofascia consists of more loosely woven fibers compared to dense tissues such as tendons and ligaments.

Myofascia is like a citrus fruit. If you cut a grapefruit in half, you'll see the juicy part of the fruit is contained in tiny sacks, and those tiny sacks are contained within larger sacks that you scoop out to eat, and so on. In the same way, muscle tissue is contained in sacks within sacks of fascia. The layers of fascia are continuous with and integrated into the muscle's tendon, which connects to the bone (Kamrami et al. 2021).

Despite their close relationship, muscle and fascia are made of different stuff and, therefore, are responsible for different aspects of human movement.

Muscle is contractile. When a muscle contracts, it pulls on its attachment sites to create movement and returns to its resting length when it relaxes. We can think of muscle as the "active" component of the myofascial system. Because fascia (and all connective tissue) is relatively non-contractile, we can think of it as the "passive" component of the myofascial system.

To complicate matters just a tiny bit, fibroblast cells that produce collagen can differentiate into myofibroblasts, which actually do contract to create tension across their surrounding connective tissue (Schleip et al. 2012). This cellular contraction is especially important in the process of wound healing as it helps mend tissues together after injury (Kendall and Feghall-Bostwick 2014).

Some theorize that impaired behavior of fibroblasts and myofibroblasts in bendy people's connective tissue could be associated with the slower wound healing and atrophic (indented or less robust) scarring in people with hypermobility syndromes (Schleip et al. 2012). So, even though connective tissue isn't *entirely* passive, it is *relatively* passive compared to muscle.

Active and passive structures work together to provide mobility and stability for human movement (Panjabi 1992). While muscle contraction generates the force for movement, connective tissues transmit that force across joints, making movement integrated and efficient (Provenzano and Vanderby 2006; Zitnay and Weiss 2018).

CONNECTIVE TISSUES UNDER LOADS

As we move around in these bodies, our tissues experience all sorts of loads. Load is any force that's exerted on the tissues (Mitchell 2019). Our bodies are exposed to a variety of loads all the time, including tensile loads (stretch), compression (hello, gravity!), and others. Additionally, our tissues respond to loads in various ways, depending on the composition of the tissues.

In the chapter "Stretching," I'll further discuss how various tissues respond to stretch. For now, I'll give you a teaser: collagen-rich connective tissue exhibits a viscoelastic response to stretching. That means when you pull on it, it changes shape, or deforms, relatively slowly (relative to muscle). The deformation of connective tissue is sometimes called "tissue creep" (Stecco 2015). Once the stretch is removed, it returns, or recoils, to its resting length relatively slowly (Stecco 2015).

Something else that may surprise you is that connective tissue adapts to loads by becoming stronger. You may be familiar with this concept when applied to bone. Wolff's Law states that normal healthy bone will adapt to the loads under which it is placed so it becomes stronger to resist those loads (Cyron and Humphrey 2017). That's why you've probably heard about the importance of weight-bearing exercise for people with osteoporosis, or brittle bones. Weight-bearing brings a mechanical load to the bone, which stimulates it to become stronger and more mineral-dense (Shanb and Youssef 2014).

Less known is Davis's Law, which states that, like bone, soft connective tissue also adapts to mechanical loads by becoming stronger and more able to withstand those loads (Cyron and Humphrey 2017). According to Davis's Law, if you expose your connective tissues to a lot of stretching, they become better able to withstand stretching. If you expose them to a lot of compression, they become better able to withstand compression.

This is a massive oversimplification of tissue behavior. Many "load parameters" would impact the specific way connective tissue adapts to loads. Load parameters include things such as frequency of the load, duration, magnitude, angle, and others (Mitchell 2019). However, understanding the basic concept will help us as we move forward to discuss what's different about connective tissue for bendy people.

WHAT'S DIFFERENT ABOUT BENDY CONNECTIVE TISSUE?

As I discussed in the chapter "Hypermobility 101," the genetic difference of bendy people's collagen structure and function (or fibroblast behavior) results in increased connective tissue laxity—something I like to call "floppiness." That means collagen fibers don't behave as much like steel cables in the bendy body.

Bendy connective tissue yields to tensile loads more easily but returns even more slowly to its resting length (Alsiri et al. 2019; Rombaut et al. 2012). In other words, it creeps more easily and stays "creeped out" for longer. This isn't the result of years of yoga practice; it's the result of genetics.

I recently had a chance to talk with Jules Mitchell—biomechanist, yoga instructor, and author of *Yoga Biomechanics: Stretching Redefined*. Her book is a fascinating look at many things relevant to yoga asana practice, including connective tissue behavior. In our conversation about yoga and hypermobility, she emphasized:

> Tissue laxity means the tissue has less ability to recoil. Connective tissue is extremely resilient, but everybody has different connective tissue properties genetically. You cannot reverse tissue laxity in somebody with hypermobility because that is in the genetic makeup; it's a result of the way fibroblasts are making collagen. You can do all the yoga you want, and if you don't have a genetic disposition for it, you're not going to get hypermobility. It's not something you can catch. Yoga doesn't cause hypermobility; yoga self-selects for people with hypermobility.

Even though bendy people have more tissue laxity, that doesn't mean their tissues can't adapt to loads. Research suggests that they can indeed become stronger, more resilient, and better able to withstand loads (Moller et al. 2014; Palmer et al. 2020). Understanding how to create optimal adaptation for bendy connective tissue is largely person-specific and far beyond the scope of this book. For now, you can trust that a bendy person is capable of improving their tissues' tolerance to loads, even if it requires the guidance and monitoring of a qualified professional.

WHY DO WE CARE?

The unique qualities of bendy connective tissue directly impact how bendy people experience yoga asana. Earlier in the chapter, I discussed active and passive components of the myofascial system and explained how connective tissue transmits the force of muscular contraction across joints for integrated and efficient movement.

The tension (or tautness) of connective tissue is what helps it transmit force (Zitnay and Weiss 2018). Now, imagine what it might be like if all your connective tissue was floppy. Floppy fascia, floppy ligaments, floppy joint capsules...you get the idea.

Floppy connective tissue can't transmit force across joints as effectively, leading to movement inefficiency and muscle fatigue. If you're a bendy yoga practitioner who seems to fatigue more easily than your peers, this could be one reason why.

Impaired force transmission also has a surprising impact on the sensory function of connective tissue. Connective tissues are full of specialized nerve cells called mechanoreceptors which sense pressure, stretch, motion, and the position of joints (Iheanacho and Vellipuram 2021). When stimulated by a force such as tension, they send information to the brain about what's going on in the body.

Because bendy connective tissue is floppy, its mechanoreceptors aren't as easily stimulated. That means they're not as good at detecting and transmitting important sensory information such as pressure, stretch, motion, and joint position during movement.

During my conversation with Jules Mitchell, she brought this relationship to light:

Laxity is not a failure of the connective tissue. It's still doing its job. But connective tissue has a lot of jobs, and what's most important—in my opinion—is force transmission. When you have lax tissue, you have less force transmission. Think of all the proprioceptors [mechanoreceptors that sense the body's position] and all the other mechanical receptors that lie in and around your joints. They sense force. If you have diminished force transmission because you have lax tissue, then your proprioceptors may not be getting the mechanical stimulus they need.

Tissue laxity goes hand in hand with a decreased ability to discern and interpret sensations in the body, including proprioception. Proprioception is the ability to sense the position of the joints (and hence, the whole body) in space. It's a complex sense that also plays a role in our ability to smoothly control movement and determine the right amount of force to use for a task (Ergen and Ulkar 2007).

Decreased proprioception leaves bendy brains wondering where we are in space and potentially unaware when we are moving too far into a yoga posture and perhaps putting ourselves at risk for injury. Jules went on to say, "Teaching someone with hypermobility to sense is more important than adapting their collagen."

Connective tissue behavior is complicated. While we sometimes consider it to be purely mechanical, it is intimately tied to how we sense and experience our bodies and, therefore, the decisions we make about movement. Understanding the unique features of bendy connective tissue can inform our approach to asana practice and teaching for those with hypermobility syndromes, both from a mechanical and sensory perspective.

In the next chapter, I'll review some of the most common symptoms and comorbidities (co-occurring conditions) that people with HSD/hEDS often experience. Then in Part Two, I'll explore principles of asana practice that support their unique bodies.

CHAPTER 4:

Common Bendy Body Complaints

———

"Something that comes as a surprise to many is that up to 70 percent of people with anxiety and panic disorders have joint hypermobility."

In the chapter "Hypermobility 101," I mentioned that people with HSD/hEDS have more risk for developing a variety of musculoskeletal pain and injury (Magee 2008) as well as wide-ranging comorbidities (co-occurring conditions). In this chapter, I'll paint a picture of the most common bendy body complaints within the tangled ball of yarn we call HSD/ hEDS. Not all bendy people have all these challenges, and some have others not included here.

Rather than stoking fear in your heart about all the things that can go "wrong," let this chapter broaden your awareness about bendiness. The remainder of the book will include tips and recommendations for designing a yoga practice with these conditions, tendencies, and increased injury risks in mind.

JOINT DISLOCATION, SUBLUXATION, AND PAIN

Because bendy people have more connective tissue laxity, their ligaments and joint capsules don't offer as much stability, making them more prone to joint dislocation and subluxation (Shirley et al. 2012). Dislocation is when the two bones that form a joint separate completely, whereas subluxation describes a partial dislocation. People with severe cases of joint instability require bracing or mobility aids due to frequent dislocations during mundane tasks or even while sleeping.

The shoulder is an inherently mobile joint because the socket (glenoid fossa of the scapula) is so shallow. Although technically a "ball and socket" joint, it would be more accurate to call it a "ball-on-a-plate" joint. Hence, if a bendy person were to dislocate a joint in yoga class (let's hope they don't!), it would most likely be a shoulder.

The vast majority of shoulder dislocations—though not all—are anterior, meaning the humeral head pops forward out of the socket. Shoulder abduction to about 90 degrees out to the side with external rotation places the shoulder at most risk for anterior dislocation, particularly when it's loaded (Cutts, Steven, et al. 2009).

Sometimes the humerus pops right back in on its own after a dislocation, but usually, it needs to be "reduced," or put back in by a professional. Beware: trying to reduce your own shoulder dislocation can lead to a fracture of the humerus, so I would always seek professional help in this case.

In contrast, the hip is a relatively stable joint. However, hip dysplasia, a congenital condition that leads to a shallow socket, is much more prevalent among those with hypermobility and increases the risk of hip dislocation (Muldoon et al. 2016).

During pregnancy, joints become less stable due to the hormone relaxin. Relaxin softens ligaments and joint capsules so the pelvis can expand during childbirth. During pregnancy, it increases the risk for generalized joint hypermobility and the injury risk that comes along with that. For a bendy person who is also pregnant, this is a double whammy.

If someone has a history of joint instability or dislocation, it would be wise for them to get guidance from their doctor or physical therapist before practicing asana.

Joint pain is a common complaint among bendy people, but, in particular, sacroiliac joint pain tops the charts (Beijk et al. 2021; Ali et al. 2020). It is the number one complaint I hear from bendy yoga practitioners. It's usually characterized by a sharpish localized pain on one side or the other near the top of the sacrum. It's thought to be the result of relatively decreased stability and increased shear strain in the sacroiliac joint.

Temporomandibular (jaw) Joint Dysfunction (TMD) is another commonly-reported challenge for bendy people (Kavuncu et al. 2006).

LABRAL TEARS

Shoulder and hip joints have an extra ring of cartilage called a labrum surrounding the joint socket. The labrum deepens the socket for more stability. When torn, the joint has less stability. Labral tears are not always a problem; in fact, research shows many people have labral tears in their hips or shoulders without any symptoms (Register et al. 2012). If a labral tear is symptomatic, it is most often exacerbated by end-range movements.

I've worked with more than a few bendy yoga practitioners who have suspected hip labral tears or show signs of femoroacetabular impingement. Femoroacetabular impingement describes the hip labrum getting pinched between the femur and the hip socket. It's most likely to occur when the hip is flexed (thigh toward the chest), abducted (out to the side), and externally rotated, which is the position of the hip in postures many refer to as "hip openers" (Groh and Herrera 2009).

SPRAINS AND STRAINS

Sprain and strain are commonly used interchangeably, but they have different meanings. "Sprain" refers to a ligament injury (Magee 2008). Ligaments connect bone to bone and help reinforce joints for more stability. Ankle sprain is a classic example in which an ankle ligament is overstretched or ruptured. Unfortunately, ligament injuries take a long time to heal, and they lead to more instability and decreased proprioception (joint position sense) for the affected joint.

"Strain" refers to an injury of muscle or tendon. Tendons connect muscles to bone. A strain may occur due to a sudden strong muscle contraction or stretching the muscle to the point of injury (Magee 2008).

When a tendon is irritated, inflamed, or painful, we refer to it as "tendinitis." Common examples of tendinitis are tennis elbow (lateral epicondylitis) and rotator cuff tendinitis of the shoulder. When tendon irritation becomes chronic, meaning it persists for longer than eight to twelve weeks, it's usually referred to as "tendinopathy" (Hicks 2020).

Bendy people tend to get a lot of sprains and strains. It can be hard to keep up with them. One week it's the elbow, the next, it's the knee, and so on. Sprains and strains are most likely to occur at end ranges of motion during asana practice or during fast-paced movement that's not well controlled. For someone with frequent strains and sprains, one-on-one attention from a professional is recommended.

HEADACHES

Chronic headache is one of the most common complaints of people with HSD/hEDS. The causes are many.

People with HSD/hEDS are more likely to have a Chiari Malformation (Milhorat et al. 2007) in which the bottom portion
of the brain bulges through the large hole at the bottom of the
skull. Chiari Malformation can lead to a variety of potential
problems in addition to headaches, such as difficulty with
swallowing, breathing, hearing, and balance (NINDS 2022).

Spontaneous cerebrospinal fluid leak is also more likely to
occur in a bendy body. This is a condition in which the mem-
branes surrounding the brain and spinal cord, which are
made of connective tissue, rupture and allow fluid to leak out.

Not surprisingly, bendy people are more likely to have
craniocervical instability, which is to say the joints at the
top of their neck are extra wobbly. This leads to compensatory neck muscle tension and is also a contributing factor for
Chiari Malformation (Milhorat et al. 2007).

PELVIC FLOOR, GYNECOLOGICAL, AND REPRODUCTIVE CHALLENGES

Pelvic Organ Prolapse (POP) is so common for bendy people
that it's one of the diagnostic criteria for hEDS. POP is when
the bladder, rectum, uterus, or even the intestines, pushes
into the vagina from the inside and starts to move down
and out of the body. Stress urinary incontinence—loss of
urine during activities like sneezing, coughing, running, and
jumping—is also common for bendy people (Gilliam et al.
2020).

Optimal function of the pelvic floor muscles is important for both conditions. A bendy person's pelvic floor muscles are likely to be tense or chronically contracted in addition to being relatively weak. Pelvic floor muscle tension can lead to pelvic pain, pain with intercourse, or even chronic constipation (Gilliam et al. 2020). These complaints warrant a trip to a pelvic physical therapist.

People with hypermobility syndromes have been shown to have a higher prevalence of heavy or prolonged menstrual bleeding, severe menstrual cramping, painful intercourse, and more frequent pregnancy loss (Hugon-Rodin et al. 2016). And for many young people, the hormonal changes that come with puberty initiate or worsen their hypermobility syndrome symptoms.

DYSAUTONOMIA

Dysautonomia describes dysfunction of the autonomic nervous system leading to difficulty regulating heart rate, blood pressure, and other basic functions. Dysautonomia is a broad umbrella term and may include a variety of manifestations. The most common way this shows up for those with HSD/ hEDS is Postural Orthostatic Tachycardia Syndrome (POTS), when the heart rate elevates more and stays elevated for longer than normal upon standing.

Symptoms of POTS include heart palpitations, fatigue, exercise intolerance, brain fog, and dizziness. It can make being upright quite uncomfortable. The technical term for this is Orthostatic Intolerance. Research has shown up to 80 percent of people with hypermobility syndromes have Orthostatic Intolerance (Gazit et al. 2003; Csecs et al. 2020), and other research has found joint hypermobility in up to 70 percent of patients with POTS (Mathias et al. 2012).

Bendy people tend to have low blood pressure, commonly attributed to their saggy blood vessels, which can't maintain adequate tension (pressure) in the system. Increased heart rate upon standing is one way the body compensates for low blood pressure.

Saggy vessels allow blood to pool in the lower body, which can impair blood flow to the brain and contribute to brain fog and fatigue. Neck pain and headaches are also strongly associated with POTS (Mack et al. 2010). Decreased blood flow to the neck and upper back muscles is thought to contribute to these complaints (Khurana 2012).

POTS can contribute to impaired exercise tolerance, in which people are more easily winded during exercise or have significant fatigue and muscle soreness following exercise (Maya et al. 2021).

Milder cases of POTS can often be ameliorated with progressive training to improve orthostatic tolerance and cardiovascular fitness. For someone with a severe case of POTS, this should be done with the guidance of a doctor or physical therapist.

MENTAL HEALTH AND NEURODEVELOPMENTAL DIFFERENCES

Anxiety is one of the most common mental health challenges among bendy people (Bulbena et al. 1993; Martin-Santos et al. 1998). Up to 70 percent of people with anxiety and panic disorders demonstrate joint hypermobility (Eccles et al. 2012).

Increased autonomic reactivity linked to differences in brain structure is thought to underly this phenomenon. People with hypermobility have larger amygdalae than their non-bendy counterparts (Eccles et al. 2012). The amygdala is part of the brain involved in fear and threat detection and is related to a person's response to danger. Moreover, when exposed to emotional stimuli, hypermobile people show increased reactivity in their amygdala and other areas of the brain involved with emotional processing and autonomic regulation (Eccles et al. 2016).

Hypermobility has also been shown to be significantly more prevalent in populations with a variety of neurodevelopmental conditions (Casanova et al. 2020; Csecs et al. 2020). In 2020, Csecs et al. found that joint hypermobility is over four times more prevalent among people with Autism Spectrum Disorder and ADHD compared to controls, and about seven times more prevalent among those with Tourette's Syndrome (Csecs et al. 2020). Other research has also found a strong association between joint hypermobility and adult ADHD (Glans et al. 2021).

ALTERED INTEROCEPTION

Interoception is the ability to sense physiological states, such as hunger, thirst, or the need to urinate. It includes changes in heart rate and blood pressure and the presence of muscle tension. The sensations related to changing emotional states are also considered to be interoceptive signals.

People with hypermobility have been shown to have a heightened sensitivity to interoceptive signals, which is correlated with dysautonomia (Eccles et al. 2012). It's like the volume dial on their interoception is turned up. This can make it difficult to discern and interpret inner sensations. In addition, many bendy people have increased sensitivity to sound, light, or other sensory stimuli, and many have difficulty integrating sensory experience.

Bendy people's heightened interoceptive sensitivity may, in part, explain the association between hypermobility and neurodevelopmental differences mentioned above (Eccles et al. 2014). Research also demonstrates a strong association between bendy people's interoceptive sensitivity and anxiety (MallorquÃ-BaguÃ et al. 2014).

Many people consider heightened interoceptive sensitivity to be a gift as well as a challenge. In fact, some interesting research suggests people with increased interoceptive sensitivity are more altruistic and tend toward more generosity with others (Piech et al. 2017).

IMPAIRED PROPRIOCEPTION

It's not uncommon for bendy people to report feeling clumsy—this is consistent with the well-documented struggle bendy people have with proprioception, the ability to sense joint and body position in space (Clayton et al. 2015). There are a couple of reasons for the struggle. As I discussed in the chapter "Connective Tissue Nitty-Gritty," floppy connective tissue doesn't get the sensory stimulation it needs to effectively transmit mechanical information, including joint position, to the brain.

In addition, some fascinating research has shown bendy people have a smaller parietal cortex than their non-bendy counterparts. The parietal cortex, where the somatosensory cortex is located in the brain, receives sensory information from the body. Every part of the body is mapped out within the somatosensory cortex such that sensory information from your right hand travels directly to the "right hand" part of the map, and so on. Having less body-mapping real estate is thought to contribute to decreased sensory awareness, poor proprioception, and lack of coordination (Eccles et al. 2012).

MUSCLE TENSION

One of the top complaints of bendy people is the feeling of muscle tension and pain (Tinkle 2020), and it's one of the things that draws bendy people to yoga. The feeling of tension is a highly subjective experience. But there are several reasons why a bendy person's muscles might be chronically contracted, fatigued, and cranky.

A bendy person's muscular system must work over time to compensate for the lack of stability from connective tissues such as ligaments, joint capsules, and fascia. The only way a muscle knows how to do that is to contract, which could lead to chronic muscle contraction and fatigue.

Common postural impairments are also problematic for bendy people because they can further trigger chronic muscular contraction. Chronically contracted muscles don't get adequate blood flow, so cellular waste products aren't flushed out as effectively. You end up with what I call "a painful chemical soup," causing irritation in the tissue (Hallman and Lyskov 2012).

Dysautonomia (see above) can also play a role in muscle tension. In response to low blood pressure and volume that results from saggy or leaky blood vessels, the sympathetic nervous system has to turn things up a notch to maintain adequate blood pressure and heart rate. On top of that, bendy people's enlarged and hyper-reactive amygdala also increases sympathetic arousal. Unfortunately, sympathetic arousal leads to increased muscle tension (Hallman and Lyskov 2012).

FIBROMYALGIA

Fibromyalgia is a chronic pain condition characterized by widespread tenderness throughout the body and is often associated with fatigue, brain fog, and sleep disturbance, among other symptoms. It is thought to be related to a hypersensitized nervous system that generates a pain response even when one isn't warranted (Boomershine 2015).

Pain is complex, but in the simplest terms, pain is the brain's alarm system. Your brain sets off the alarm system when it senses tissue damage or threat. In response to an acute injury such as burning your hand, your brain generates pain to tell you to protect your injury so it can heal. Most tissues in the body heal within eight to twelve weeks. Pain that persists beyond normal tissue healing time is called chronic or persistent pain.

Most cases of chronic pain, including fibromyalgia, are thought to be the result of a broken pain alarm system in which the nervous system becomes hypersensitive, hypervigilant, and falls into a habit of generating a pain response even in the absence of tissue damage. The pain isn't any less real; it just isn't well explained by tissue damage. Research has found a whopping 80 percent of patients with fibromyalgia have joint hypermobility (Eccles et al. 2021).

CHRONIC FATIGUE SYNDROME AND SLEEP DISTURBANCE

Chronic Fatigue Syndrome (CFS) is a condition of extreme fatigue that persists for over six months, is not relieved by rest, and isn't explained by any other medical condition (Mayo Foundation 2022). It is also sometimes called Myalgic Encephalomyelitis (ME). This condition is common among people with HSD/hEDS (The Ehlers-Danlos Society 2022; Hakim et al. 2017). Symptoms typically include brain fog, post-exertional malaise (feeling even worse after physical activity), difficulty with concentration and memory, and dizziness (Mayo Foundation 2022).

Even in the absence of CFS/ME, sleep is a common struggle for bendy people in general (Moss et al. 2018). Dysautonomia is one contributing factor. Many people with POTS (Postural Orthostatic Tachycardia Syndrome), which is the most common form of dysautonomia for bendy people, experience intermittent adrenaline surges that can cause frequent waking during the night (Cleveland Clinic 2022). Of course, sleep is critical to overall well-being and to maintaining energy for the activities that help you feel better, including a well-designed yoga practice.

MAST CELL ACTIVATION DISORDER AND AUTOIMMUNITY

Mast cells are one of your immune system's first lines of defense. They release histamine and other inflammatory mediators in response to allergens. Mast Cell Activation Disorder (MCAD) is when mast cells release their inflammatory molecules even when they shouldn't, leading to skin rashes and hives, especially in response to stress, heat, or exercise. It is also associated with a host of other symptoms, including brain fog, lightheadedness, flushing, stomach pain, and others. MCAD is common for people with HSD/hEDS, even though the relationship between them is not well understood (Kohn and Chang 2020).

People with hEDS also have a higher prevalence of autoimmune conditions, including Rheumatoid Arthritis and Ankylosing Spondylitis, compared with the general population (Rodgers et al. 2017; Makol et al. 2021). Some research has also shown a higher-than-normal correlation between EDS and Multiple Sclerosis (Vilisaar et al. 2008), and even that HSD symptoms can mimic those of MS (Riggs et al. 2018). Again, these relationships are not yet well understood.

DIGESTIVE DISORDERS AND DISORDERED EATING

Whether it's Irritable Bowel Syndrome (IBS), chronic constipation, or leaky gut, bendy people have a range of digestive system issues (Fikree et al. 2017). Many have food sensitivities that require restrictive diets (Cutts, R.M. et al. 2012). Working with a doctor or nutritionist to determine the most effective approach to diet and supplementation is recommended.

Hypermobility has been correlated with a higher prevalence of eating disorders (Baeza-Velasco et al. 2022). Some research suggests that up to 63 percent of people with Anorexia Nervosa have joint hypermobility, and over 50 percent have POTS—one of the most common comorbidities in hypermobility syndromes (Goh et al. 2013). Some research also shows interoceptive sensitivity and the misinterpretation of interoceptive signals is strongly associated with Anorexia Nervosa (Jacquemot and Park 2020).

SUMMARY

From joint injury to dysautonomia to fatigue and so much more, the challenges associated with HSD/hEDS can impact yoga practice in a variety of ways. Many practitioners will benefit from asana modifications or alternative positioning, and they will likely respond more favorably to certain breathing practices versus others. A broad understanding of

HSD/hEDS will help us approach yoga practice in a way that supports the unique needs of bendy people.

While mindfulness is warranted, it's not helpful to be overly cautious with people who have hypermobility syndromes. Despite its differences, the bendy body is strong and adaptable, and the benefits of asana practice far outweigh the risks in the vast majority of cases.

In the next chapter, I'll unpack the most common question I get about yoga and hypermobility, namely: "Is yoga bad for bendy people?" Then, in Parts Two and Three, I will make specific recommendations for how bendy people can avoid the most common injuries and instead find support through yoga practice. My recommendations will relate directly back to what you have learned in this chapter.

CHAPTER 5:

Is Yoga Bad for Bendy People?

"There's no need to throw the baby out with the bathwater, as they say."

It may come as no surprise that bendy people love yoga. With all the positive feedback they get for their natural ability to achieve complicated postures, it's easy to understand the attraction. Other students often gaze with envy at the hyper-mobile student getting easily into pretzel shapes, wishing they too had such an ease of movement.

I've heard countless hypermobile yoga practitioners tell me yoga was the first physical activity they ever felt good at. Many of them report finding a sense of physical mastery for the first time. It sometimes seems yoga asana is nearly irresistible for hypermobile people. So, let's get back to our question, "Is yoga bad for bendy people?"

You'll get a range of answers to this question depending on who you ask. But when people ask this, they are actually asking, "Is yoga *asana*—the physical practice of postures—bad for bendy people?"

Some well-meaning doctors and physical therapists argue people with hypermobility should stay away from yoga asana because the risk of injury is too great.

Kerry Gabrielson is an attorney living with hEDS and the host of the *Hypermobility Happy Hour Podcast*, which raises awareness about hypermobility syndromes. In a recent conversation I had with her, she shared the unfortunate advice she received from her doctor upon her hEDS diagnosis in 2016:

> I started doing yoga a few years before I was diagnosed. I didn't know about hypermobility, and I often had aches and pains after class. But overall, it was very beneficial. I was in the best shape of my life. I felt strong, had more defined muscle mass, and slept better. When I was diagnosed in 2016, that doctor told me to stop doing yoga because it was too much of a risk for my joints and I would just be doing more damage to them. When I stopped, I de-conditioned pretty rapidly, and my symptoms went downhill.

Kerry's doctor's limited understanding led him to dismiss a practice that was actually serving her for the most part. On the other end of the spectrum are others, usually starry-eyed yoga teachers committed to their version of yoga asana being *the right thing* for everyone, who argue all this worry about injury for bendy people is unfounded.

My answer is, "Well, it depends." As I mentioned in my Introduction, the devil is in the details. In some cases, asana practice can certainly lead to injury for bendy people. As Dr. Linda Bluestein reflected in our recent conversation, "I definitely have lots of patients who say, 'I got hurt in yoga,' or 'I got hurt by doing yoga.'"

But there are many styles of asana practice. Some are likely to be more conducive to injury than others. Some styles of asana are form-centric, meaning they are primarily concerned with your body's specific position in yoga postures. Other styles are breath-centric, meaning they are primarily concerned with some quality of the breath during an asana practice. Some involve propping yourself up on soft squishy bolsters and relaxing deeply for the entire class. Others involve performing challenging postures while you sweat in a heated room. Some move quickly; others move slowly.

Claims about the benefits of x, y, or z type of asana practice are everywhere. It's quite the norm for yoga teachers to proclaim their style of asana as the "be-all and end-all" and that it's right for everyone. Various types of practice are described as "therapeutic" or touted as being "healing for the knees" and so on. These claims are based on a key assumption that we all have the same needs. Labeling a particular type of asana practice as "therapeutic" assumes what's therapeutic for you is also therapeutic for me and, likewise, for everyone else. This is not the case.

Let's assume twenty people do an asana practice advertised as therapeutic. Let's assume ten of them feel amazing after class (awesome!), five feel about the same (we'll take it!), and the other five feel agitated or have more pain (bummer). If those last five people expected a positive effect but instead had a negative effect, how should they make sense of this dissonance?

They typically assume they did something wrong. What ensues is a continued effort at doing the same type of practice *more correctly* or with *better alignment* until they get the expected results. Expecting everyone to benefit from the same type of asana practice is a problem. A focus on external expectations leads practitioners to override or ignore cues from their bodies and instead put their trust in others who claim to know better. This leads to disempowerment for all practitioners, but it's particularly unhelpful for bendy people who tend to have difficulty understanding their body's cues as it is.

When we replace external expectations with an inquiry into our inner experience of asana, we gain the freedom to notice our unique response to a practice just as it is. That's where transformation begins.

Maria Morrin is a bendy yoga teacher in Ireland. In a recent conversation I had with her, she recounted her experience of a yin yoga class in 2019. Although not all yin yoga classes are the same, yin yoga is typically characterized by long (3–5 minute) stretches held in a relaxed way at end range. Maria had never been to a yin yoga class before, but she was intrigued.

When she arrived at the class, she remembers hearing other students chatting about how great they felt after the previous week's class and, specifically, how much energy they had afterward. The teacher even chimed in to say yes, indeed, yin yoga is so energizing that she often goes home and cleans her house from top to bottom after practice. Well, for Maria, who had long struggled with the chronic fatigue commonly associated with hypermobility, the thought of leaving class energized for the rest of the day was exciting.

> I was sitting there thinking, "Wow! If this practice could fill me with energy, that would be amazing!" I was getting excited about how my afternoon might go, because I was about to do something that was going to make me feel really good.

Maria made her way through the class with no problems. When class was over, she waved goodbye and headed out to her car. Then she describes a response to the practice that was anything but what she was expecting. As she got into her car, a wave of profound fatigue washed over her.

> I thought, "Okay, maybe I'm just gonna feel tired for a bit before all the energy arrives." I came home and my partner asked, "How'd your class go?" and I was like, "I need to go to bed right now." I literally just collapsed in exhaustion and slept for a few hours.

Maria and I discussed how it felt to encounter dissonance between externalized expectations and the reality of her own experience. She described how she went over many options in her mind for how to explain how she felt after class and how disappointing it was that she didn't feel the same way everyone else seemed to feel.

I remember trying to reason it in my mind, thinking, "Maybe it's toxins released from the muscles after stretching, and I need to drink more water?" But I couldn't help wondering, "If everyone else feels so good after this practice, why am I completely wiped?" And then I felt disappointed and a bit sorry for myself because I thought, "Here's another supposedly great practice that doesn't work for me."

The key point here isn't whether yin yoga is bad for bendy people. The key point is simply about the dangers of setting up expectations for how people should respond to any specific type of practice.

In Maria's case, several reasons may explain why she was exhausted rather than energized by the class. Maybe it was just going to be an exhausted kind of day regardless of what she did. Maybe all that passive end-range stretching left her nervous system feeling a bit out of whack (see the chapter "Stretching"). Maybe after stretching her already-floppy connective tissues, her body required more muscular effort to hold her body together (yawn).

Maria describes how that experience informs her teaching and how she routinely gives students permission to be as they are rather than as they expect to be.

Just last night I was teaching a vigorous breath practice in class, and I said, "You may feel energized after this, or your body's response to it might be quite different, but however you feel, it's perfectly valid. There's no one prescription that's going to make everyone feel a certain way, you can only discover how it makes you feel today."

Many well-meaning yoga teachers like to claim their style of asana practice is great for everyone. But a practice has no merit or fault on its own. It is simply a certain approach to, or series of, postures and other techniques. It takes on meaning when someone practices it. Then the question becomes about the practitioner, not the practice. It's not so helpful to ask, "Is this a good practice?" The more helpful question is, "Is this a good practice *for this specific practitioner?*"

In other words, what does the practitioner need based on injury history, goals, and other factors, and does this practice help meet those needs? Moreover, does this practice lead the practitioner closer to the ultimate aims of yoga? It's reasonable to expect a room full of yoga practitioners to have a wide variety of responses to the same practice.

When there's a match between a practice and the needs of a practitioner, it can be a healing, integrating experience. But, when there's a mismatch, it can be a recipe for pain and injury. One of the gems I have gleaned from my studies in the viniyoga lineage is: All yoga practice is about the practitioner. It's never about the practice. Your job as a practitioner is to learn how to make yoga good at you rather than twisting yourself around to become "good" at yoga as if it is something outside yourself that you're striving to attain.

When it comes to bendy people, a useful question is, "What types of yoga practice are most likely to be supportive for bendy people given their unique needs?" Even though all people are unique, we can make some broad brushstrokes about the types of practices that *most likely* won't work well for those with HSD/hEDS, and the types that *most likely* will work well.

In general, an asana practice that emphasizes mobility and performance is not likely to go as well. You might be thinking, "But that's where bendy people really shine!" Yes, I know. But aside from the external validation and ego boost, that approach to practice won't likely serve the bendy practitioner and, in the worst case, may lead to strains, sprains, and other injuries.

Extreme yoga postures may be fun from an acrobatic point of view, but in the context of yoga, I'm interested in the *why*. Why include a split in your practice? What benefit does it bring, and how does it help you reach your ultimate goals? Unless you are a circus performer, it's not that useful. Life mostly happens in midranges, not at end ranges. Most of us aren't training for the circus; we're training for life.

Many years back, I had a bendy yoga-teaching patient who was struggling with a hamstring strain (pain at the hamstring attachment to the sitting bone) and sacroiliac joint pain. I worked with her to improve the recruitment, strength, and control of the muscles in the back of her body. I also suggested she give forward folding a rest. Not forever, but for a while.

Like many yoga-teaching bendy patients of mine, she was reluctant. Give forward folding a rest? Was I insane? She had wrapped her identity as a yoga teacher up in her ability to perform deep forward folds. She was at the crossroads that many bendy yoga teachers come to. She had to decide: Did she want to feel better, or did she want to look impressive in her forward folds?

She protested, "But what if I lose my range of motion?"

To which I responded, "That's a great question. What would happen if you lost some of your range of motion?"

She didn't have an answer for me, so I offered her this: "If you lose a bit of your range of motion, you'll still have more than most humans have, and nothing much about your life will have changed."

She gave a half-baked effort at the changes I suggested, but she continued to seek a different solution.

Over time, I watched as she dabbled in a variety of approaches to resolving her troubles short of changing her practice. I realized she was committed to her long-standing idea of what it means to be good at yoga. She thought if she could just do the practice more correctly or with better alignment, her problem would resolve.

Unfortunately, you can't "alignment" your way out of every-thing. If your body wants you to stop doing a certain posture, it doesn't usually matter what micro-alignment change you make. Your body still doesn't want you to do it. It's hard to give up part of a yoga practice you've been committed to. But I don't think yoga's feelings will be hurt if you eliminate a problematic posture from your practice. What inherent value does a posture have on its own, especially if it causes you pain and suffering?

This bendy yoga practitioner wasn't willing to accept that her practice wasn't the right match for her needs. I don't know if her problem ever resolved; I hope it did.

Jill Miller—yoga therapist, developer of Yoga Tune Up®, and author of *The Roll Model*— shared a powerful story with me recently about her experience as a yoga student and aspiring teacher, and the ramifications it had on her life many years later.

During her early years of study, she placed a strong emphasis on achieving extreme yoga postures, working hard to push her natural mobility to the limit. Her practice involved extremely long holds in poses like headstand, shoulder stand, splits, and deep "hip openers" such as pigeon pose. Over the years, as Jill began to understand her experience through the lens of her joint hypermobility, she recalls feeling apprehensive about the impact her early yoga practice might someday have on her body.

> I realized the way I practiced for so many years was potentially harmful for me, and that I might discover this later in life. And, of course, I have. I've had a hip surgery, and at the start of the pandemic I had my first shoulder dislocation. I didn't know that this pot of gold at the end of the rainbow of going to your potential

in yoga asana was reinforcing a weakness, rather than developing a strength. I just didn't know enough.

Jill and I shared the mixed feelings we both have about "growing up" in styles of asana that exploited hypermobility and judged success based on the chance circumstance of genetics. Despite the resulting challenges and injuries, we both agreed we wouldn't trade it for anything. That's because the yoga was still in there, and it changed both of our lives for the better. Alongside the downfalls, we found something that helped us navigate and make sense of the changing and challenging reality of life.

There's no need to throw the baby out with the bathwater, as they say. I believe yoga is ready-made to support bendy people when practiced wisely. I'll never concede that yoga is bad for bendy people, but a more meaningful question is, "How can yoga be really great for bendy people?" I'll offer my suggestions in the chapters that follow.

CHAPTER 6:

Curiosity

———

"When we bring an inquiry mindset to practice, everything changes. Suddenly the postures aren't the goal at all. They are simply tools to help us learn something about ourselves."

I remember sitting in my naturopath's office several years ago. I was somewhere in the middle of the personal medical odyssey I described in the chapter "Hypermobility 101." At the time, we weren't really getting anywhere, and I was frustrated. I was tired of feeling awful. I asked, "Is this just how I'm going to feel for the rest of my life? I mean, I've tried everything!"

My naturopath's response surprised me a bit. She replied with great kindness, "Have you? Have you tried everything?"

"Well, no. Not exactly. But it feels like I've tried everything."

"Hmm. Maybe it would be helpful to get curious. Instead of saying 'I've tried everything,' try saying, '*I wonder.* I wonder what's out there that I haven't even heard of yet!'"

She was trying to help me shift my mindset into a place that allowed for more possibilities so I wouldn't get stuck in my discouragement. Curiosity is that place. Curiosity helps us stay open to learning, discovery, and possibility. In the moment, her suggestion shifted my whole inner experience, and I felt better.

In the chapter "Is Yoga Bad for Bendy People?" I discussed some pitfalls of bringing an "expectation mindset" to asana practice. However, with a "curiosity mindset," yoga postures become tools for inquiry into the unique features and condition of one's body or the investigation of subtle sensations.

For example, while in downward-facing dog pose, I could focus on forcing my body into the exact correct shape. Or I could notice how my shoulders feel about being in full flexion, or how it feels to stretch my calf muscles by bringing my heels toward the floor. I could also notice thoughts and feelings that arise in the posture, such as judgment about my performance or anticipation for what's next. Using asana to explore and investigate my body, thoughts, and feelings is more useful than trying to get the pose "right" according to an external standard.

It's easy to get attached to external standards of what yoga postures are supposed to look like rather than what they feel like. Images of beautiful and challenging yoga postures seem to be everywhere in the media. I remember a big poster that hung on the wall of a yoga studio where I practiced many years ago. It was right by the bathroom, so I would study it longingly as I waited for my turn.

The poster featured a man in tiny shorts performing fifty or more yoga postures in super-human style. I remember thinking how cool it would be to someday be able to do all those postures correctly. I'm not sure what I thought might happen once I could. I was simply lost in a world of striving. My practice wasn't about me yet; it was still about the practice.

When we hold yoga asanas outside ourselves, like on the poster, they become things to strive for and achieve for their own sake as though our ability to perform them means something. An external orientation to asana takes our focus away from ourselves, making it more difficult to notice how the practice feels. We can lose an opportunity for reflection, understanding, and ultimately transformation.

Maria Morrin, a bendy yoga teacher in Ireland, recently shared an interesting story from her yoga teacher training a few years ago. At the time, she had already been struggling with chronic pain and other challenges related to hypermobility. She found herself in even more pain during her training modules, and she wondered if her experience was typical.

During the training, I was having to take ibuprofen regularly. I remember thinking, "How can I possibly tout the benefits of yoga when I'm in so much pain?" Stuff wasn't adding up. I thought there must be something wrong with me because everyone else looked to be in this blissful state and not in discomfort.

Maria's teacher training instructor would often ask students to demonstrate specific asanas. One afternoon, Maria was chosen to demonstrate the wheel pose, which is a full backbend. She describes how good it felt to be chosen and how she was determined to perform the pose to the best of her ability. She didn't want to let anyone down.

With her instructor and peers watching, she pushed herself up into the wheel pose and immediately felt pain in her lower back. The class was focused on the way her backbend looked from the outside. Nobody seemed curious about how it felt on the inside. The juxtaposition of her pain mixed with the cheering of her classmates put her in an odd situation.

> Instead of admitting, "This doesn't feel so good. Is there anything I could do to make it more comfortable?" I didn't question it; I remember coming back down to the ground after holding it for what felt like a long time and thinking, "Holy shit, I think I might have really hurt my back." The other students were clapping and then everyone went to try and replicate what I had done. It felt confusing. I had "succeeded" in achieving the pose, but now I was in a lot of pain.

Maria's story is a powerful illustration of the dissonance so common among hypermobile people. From the outside, her backbend drew "oohs" and "aahs" from her peers and praise from her teacher. But nobody could see how much pain she was in. What's more, nobody thought to inquire about her inner experience of the asana. The posture demonstration was presented as though it was an end in and of itself. Something to achieve. Why? Nobody ever said. For her fellow students, Maria was like the man in the tiny shorts on that poster by the bathroom of my old practice studio. Her backbend was the goal.

That moment was a missed opportunity for Maria and her classmates to learn something important. With some curiosity, they could have learned about which areas of the spine allow for the most extension needed for that posture or how the posture requires a certain range of motion in the hips, spine, and shoulders. They could have discussed the function of the posture, asking important questions like, why practice the full wheel? What do we get out of it? How can the practice of this posture help us live better lives?

Most importantly, if anyone had asked Maria how it felt to do the full wheel that day, they could have learned that we all have different experiences of postures regardless of what they look like from the outside. What your full wheel looks like doesn't tell us how you feel in the pose, but curiosity will. You may be able to do it, but like Maria, you may wish you hadn't afterward.

When we bring an inquiry mindset to practice, everything changes. Suddenly the postures aren't the goal at all. They are simply tools to help us learn something about ourselves. Asana can be an opportunity to learn about our body's patterns as well as our thought habits. For example, through practicing the side plank, we can learn about the strength differences between the right and left sides of the body. And we can notice our thoughts, feelings, and judgments about that (See Figure 6a).

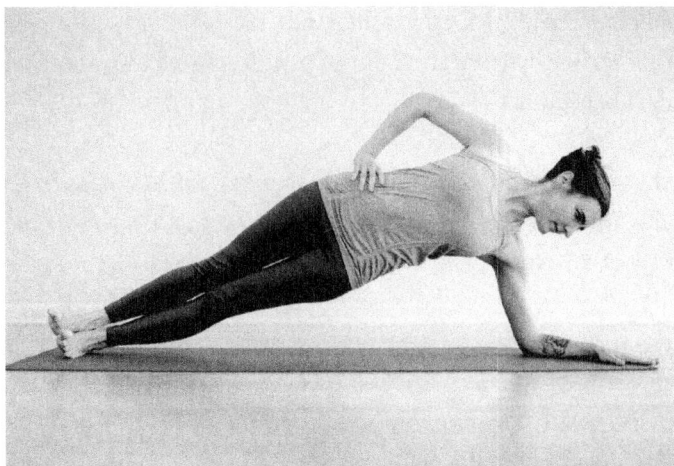

Figure 6a

When we start getting curious, we have a chance to learn about ourselves and understand more about what we need from our practice. Accordingly, we can shape our practice to meet our needs. Asana becomes a tool. It's a finger trying to point at the moon; it isn't the moon itself.

In recent years, I've gravitated toward the theme of curiosity in my teaching and practice. Curiosity carries a playfulness with it that I appreciate. I like to encourage my students to turn their attention inward with friendliness at the beginning of class and be curious about what they might learn through the practice. I invite them to study their experience, not so they can judge or fix anything, but because their inner experience is worthy of attention and can teach them something.

Unfortunately, in some yoga classes, students are actually encouraged to ignore the information from their body and instead put their trust in a teacher who claims to know better. This approach to teaching asana disempowers students by disconnecting them from their own experience.

A few years ago, I attended an asana class while traveling out of town. At the beginning of class, the instructor said something along these lines: "Even though you may think you need additional props for our practice today, I ask you to only use the props that I have suggested." Props include blankets, bolsters, straps, or blocks used to support the body in a posture. Well, right off the bat, my inner alarm was going off. I thought to myself, "Did he just ask us *not* to listen to our own bodies during this practice?" I had a feeling that things weren't going to go well, and I was right.

At one point during the practice, we were doing the reclining bound angle pose, where you lie on your back with your knees bent and feet together, then let your knees drop out to the sides. For many people, this produces a sense of stretch for the muscles of the inner thighs. We were instructed to do this posture specifically without support under our thighs for what seemed like forever.

If you've got hips like mine, there is no sensation of stretch to be found in the inner thighs in reclining bound angle pose. There is no limit to my hip range of motion other than the compression of bone on bone when the femur meets the outer rim of the hip socket at end range. That's where I was hanging out, feeling the sharp pain of compression on my outer hips, especially the left one, which had been a source of pain for many years previously.

So, there I was, desperately trying to hold my legs up to avoid resting at end range for many minutes on end. I looked longingly at the huge stack of yoga props piled up along the studio wall, a mere twenty feet away from my mat. What to do?

I was surrounded by a packed classroom. What message would it send to this room full of people if I got up and fetched the props I needed after he had explicitly asked us not to? It may have hurt his feelings, or it could have cast doubt upon his guidance for the rest of the class. So, I stayed where I was.

My body was clearly telling me what it needed. I wish I had listened. If I could go back, instead of worrying about what others would think, I'd tell myself, "This is silly. You're in charge of your body. All the time. And you need some props." It took about six months to fully resolve the hip pain flare-up caused by that one little posture in that one little class.

The yoga teacher, in this case, wasn't trying to cause me pain and suffering. He truly believed in what he was teaching. He believed the way he was instructing us to do the postures would help us somehow. Honestly, I think yoga teachers put a lot of pressure on themselves to appear knowledgeable and authoritative. And let's face it—there's something appealing about someone who has the answers. But there's a delicate balance to strike between confidence and humility. It's a balance I am always striving for as well.

At its best, the yoga teacher's role is to give students a starting point, guide them through practice, and offer suggestions and insights. Ultimately, excellent yoga teaching helps students listen inwardly, understand themselves better, and develop a positive relationship with themselves. Curiosity leads to such empowerment.

In my recent interview with Judith Hanson Lasater, we talked about how asana practice can help us learn to listen inwardly. She shared:

> Sometimes if we are doing a seated forward bend, for example, I will say to my students, "I want you to slow everything down, and I want you just to breathe. I want you to bend forward, and the very first moment you feel the slightest beginning of resistance, stop. Simply stop and don't push. Breathe and wait for the body to respond."

> Ask your body what it wants instead of telling it. Wait where you are and feel the resistance. Just wait with patience and gratitude and love. If and when the resistance dissolves, the body has answered your question. It is ready to go farther. Then maybe you slowly bend a couple more inches, but slowly, and you never ever push past resistance.

> The mind is fast. The body is slow. That's why we get injured. The mind is running the body too fast. My approach is to ask, "How can I listen with soft ears? How can I listen with softness and awareness to what the body is telling me it wants to do so I work with the speed of my body?"

It's difficult to cultivate a subtle inner awareness and listen with soft ears to the information coming from within the body. It's even more difficult to do this when you're surrounded by external cues to go farther or to achieve a certain aesthetic in a posture. Add to that a baseline deficit in proprioception (joint position sense and body awareness) that bendy people typically have, and the challenge is exponentially magnified.

In my recent interview with Dr. Linda Bluestein, she echoed this idea. She encourages her patients to approach their bodies in the same way.

I tell patients all the time, "It's listening to your body with the right ear. And also, it's listening to your body with a sense of curiosity and not letting the anxiety that so many of us feed into as you become aware of different sensations."

Just like my naturopath shifted my experience by encouraging me to say, "*I wonder...,*" I'd like to encourage you to get curious. If you're a practitioner, you have an opportunity to bring a different type of inner listening to your practice. With an attitude of curiosity, asana practice can become a place for learning about yourself.

If you're a teacher, you have an opportunity to shift your students' experience of yoga and ultimately of themselves. Do you want students to perform, or do you want to empower them to learn about themselves? If you choose the latter, your language must reflect the value of curiosity and set the tone for inquiry. I'll discuss this more in the chapter "Language and Verbal Cues."

I invite you to bring your curiosity along with you as we dive into Part Two to explore aspects of asana practice to support bendy people. We will start by exploring smaller and slower movements, various approaches to stretching, and the benefits of stability and postural awareness. Then, we will discuss how to design an asana practice and make wise use of verbal cues and hands-on assists with the needs of bendy people in mind.

PART 2:

ASANA FOR BENDY PEOPLE

CHAPTER 7:

Smaller and Slower Movements

"Just because someone can do a thing, doesn't mean they should."

In the next few chapters, I'll explore specific considerations for asana practice to ensure bendy practitioners get the most out of it. These include smaller and slower movements, varying approaches to stretching, and the benefits of stability and postural awareness. Let's begin by exploring smaller and slower movements.

Bendy bodies have a hard time setting boundaries around movement. Because their floppy connective tissue doesn't limit range of motion very well, their joints easily move all the way to end range without anything slowing them down. Their decreased proprioception (sense of joint position and body awareness) makes it more difficult to control their movements and know when they've gone far enough. Smaller and slower movements can help bendy people develop movement boundaries and improve motor control.

ASANA AS MOVEMENT

Some forms of asana feature static postures in which you hold the position for some length of time. Other forms are dynamic in which you move into and out of each posture several times or move from one posture to the next. Yet other forms of asana combine some static and some dynamic postures.

Many people think of yoga postures as static shapes that are easily defined rather than thinking of them as movements. Hence, we know the starting point and the end point, but we don't always appreciate the in-between places within a posture.

There is so much to explore about each posture if we get curious about it. For example, let's consider a high lunge. Most of us have a habitual way of practicing this posture with the front knee bent to 90 degrees. However, when we invite curiosity and inquiry, we can explore how it feels to bend the knee to varying degrees (See Figures 7a–7c). We may notice different muscle engagement in the front leg, different amounts of stretch for the back leg, and a different sense of stability and groundedness at different points.

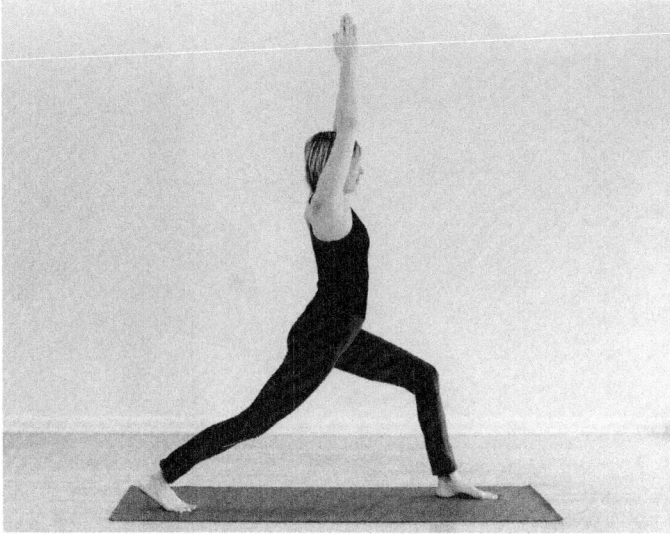

Figure 7a

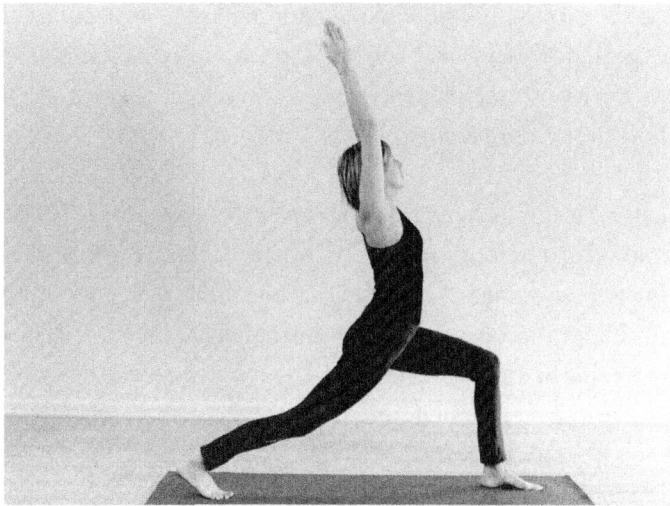

Figure 7b

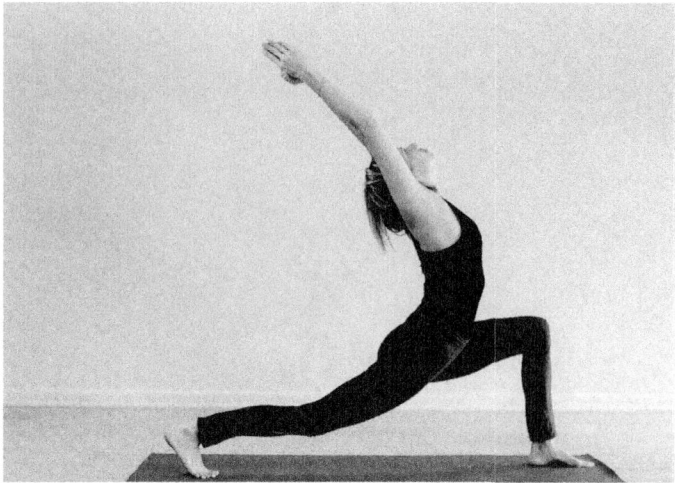
Figure 7c

If we consider postures to be fluid movements rather than static shapes, we'll see that, as it turns out, there are many versions of each one. Each version will give us a different experience. If we want to explore the in-between places within a posture, we have to let go of our expectations about how the posture is supposed to look.

Letting go of the outward appearance of a posture challenges many yoga practitioners' self-concept. I have worked with many bendy yoga practitioners who simply weren't willing to change their ways even if it meant feeling better. It's hard to be able to do a thing—especially an *impressive* thing—and still decide not to do it.

I recently had a conversation with Stepfanie Romine, a bendy yoga teacher and author living in Germany. She echoed this sentiment as she reflected on how her practice has changed over time to better support her needs.

I have so many pictures of myself in my twenties and thirties, pushing my body to its limit—doing the splits, feet behind the head, and all that. I'm so grateful I've never been seriously injured, but I've had a lot of minor injuries, little aches and pains. They taught me so much about my body. They taught me to listen and to slow down. But still, it is so hard for my ego to know that I can do more but that doing more is not beneficial.

Just because someone can do a thing, doesn't mean they should. Just because I can do a crazy deep backbend doesn't mean it serves me in any way. In fact, deep backbends make my back hurt. In general, when I contain my movement somewhere before I get to end range, my body is much happier.

SMALLER MOVEMENT

In the chapter "Hypermobility 101," I discussed that within a joint's full range of motion, there are midranges and end ranges. Keeping joints within the midrange of motion does a couple of things. It prevents joint dislocation for those prone to it and optimizes motor control. Motor control is the ability of your brain and body to communicate such that movement is purposeful, regulated, and well-coordinated (Shumway-Cook and Woollacott 2007). Think of it as stability in motion.

I've heard some yoga teachers argue excessive range of motion isn't a problem in and of itself; instead, lack of motor control within that range is what sets bendy people up for injury. So, which is it? The answer is a bit complicated.

For all bodies, motor control and joint position are related. Our ability to control movement naturally declines at end ranges. That's because muscles change length as joints move. Muscles can produce the most force (they are strongest) at midranges, reflecting a property known as the "force-length" relationship (Rassier et al. 1999). A muscle that is very short or very long can't produce as much force as one that is at mid-length.

Let's take hip flexion as an example. Hip flexion is when you move your thigh toward your chest. A handful of muscles located in the front of the hip, known as hip flexors, perform this movement. They are able to produce the best muscle contraction when the hip is in mid-range flexion. That would be anywhere from about neutral (standing) to about 90 degrees (sitting), give or take. When the hip is extended (your leg is back behind you) or deeply flexed (knees to chest), the hip flexors can't produce as much force.

Due to impaired proprioception (sense of joint position and body awareness), motor control is a common challenge for bendy people. I rarely see a person with hypermobility who is able to control movement well in midranges, much less at end range. But once good motor control can be established in midranges, then over time, we can learn to maintain control through progressively larger ranges of motion.

In most cases, it doesn't serve people with hypermobility to ever hang out at end range. However, some people actually *are* circus performers. Because performance is their goal, it makes sense for circus artists, dancers, and others to train for stability in extreme ranges so they can optimally control movement and protect their joints while they perform. But even for circus performers, stability begins with midranges and expands from there.

Sarah Blunkosky is a bendy yoga teacher and practitioner in Fredericksburg, Virginia who told me recently about the extreme joint ranges of motion she used to go into in her asana practice. She shared how grateful she is to have had excellent yoga teachers who encouraged her to cultivate stability and gentleness with her body to avoid potential long-term damage. As she shared:

> There is an epidemic in yogaland of people getting hip replacements at ages that you would not wish on anybody. I don't do deep pigeon anymore for that reason. I have no natural limits in that pose. I used to do some wacky crazy stuff in pigeon, but I've had to learn to "baby gate" myself to create my own limits. It's really kind of weird putting up artificial boundaries. I'm the one in class taking the alternative option that feels safer and will save my hip. That wonderful internal voice pops on to say, "Hey, this is enough. This gentle, supported pigeon is just as valuable as the pigeon you were doing years ago, which was kind of fun but at the same time, a great path to a hip replacement."

In my recent conversation with Jill Miller, yoga therapist and author of *The Roll Model*, we talked about the importance of developing control in midranges. She shared how she wished she'd been encouraged to explore the in-between places in yoga postures earlier in her yoga experience:

Often, hypermobile people need to hear things that nobody has been brave enough to tell them like, "Mid-range is sexy. Let's work in the gray zone, not the end zone." Those are things that would have been great if somebody had helped me with.

In asana practice, I generally recommend that bendy people intentionally back away from their end ranges to create movement boundaries and work on motor control. This means stopping a movement before you get to end range, even when your body hasn't put on the brakes. Instead, go to about 80 percent (or experiment with other amounts) of what's available.

It is usually challenging for bendy people to determine when they've gotten to 80 percent of their available range. That's when external feedback can be really helpful. Seeing their bodies in the mirror can help them determine how much movement they've done. Feedback from an instructor can also help. Over time with practice, they'll be better able to sense the amount of movement without external feedback.

Exploring the gray zone is difficult if you're moving quickly. If you want to tune in and really get to know what it feels like to move through a smaller range of motion, slowing down is key. Without slowing down, we risk missing the gray zone completely.

Slower Movement

Many bendy yoga practitioners are so accustomed to moving quickly from one end range to another without control that it can feel completely different for them to slow down. When I started exploring smaller and slower movements in asana practice, I was shocked to discover all the variety of sensations I'd always blown right past on my way to end range. I had no idea that if I just went *less far* and learned to pay attention, I would find a whole new world of sensation that I'd previously missed.

During the ten years when I had a chronic hamstring strain, I never felt a sense of stretch in my hamstring muscles when I did a forward fold. My body just kept going and going until I landed at my end range. What I felt there was a sharp pain at the place where the hamstring tendon attaches to the ischial tuberosity (sitting bone), and afterward, I always hurt worse. I never felt a sense of stretch across the length of my hamstring muscles.

Slowing down allowed me time to pay close attention to the subtle sensations I had missed by transitioning so quickly from one posture to the next. I had to investigate the in-between places to find the first hints of stretch arising in my body as I moved into yoga postures. I practiced stopping right where I felt the first hints.

I also learned to interpret the sensations that would arise when I was going too far. For example, the sensation would change in a certain way or move out of the muscle belly and toward the attachment site. I could still go farther, but I learned to stay put. When I did, asana practice didn't make my pain worse anymore. Slowing down helped me grow my sensory awareness. It also helped me build motor control.

As I shared in my introduction, the slow-moving style of asana practice I was introduced to at the Krishnamayacharya Yoga Mandiram (KYM) back in 2008 challenged me unlike any I'd ever experienced precisely because it demanded a level of physical control I simply did not have.

It may be counterintuitive but moving slowly through an asana practice is far more challenging than moving quickly. We are accustomed to a fast pace, both in yoga and in life. Momentum is easy; slow is hard. Slow requires mindfulness, curiosity, awareness, and self-control. It's no wonder that so many bendy yoga practitioners prefer fast-paced asana.

A couple of years ago, a young woman showed up to my yoga class and told me she had just been diagnosed with hEDS. Well, I was glowing on the inside, thinking she was going to fall in love with my class. I assured her that the class would be appropriate and safe for her because we move slowly and incorporate a good bit of stability work. We begin by establishing a steady breath pace and then match the pace of movement to that. It's like moving your body through honey in slow motion.

During the practice, I noticed her struggling with a simple movement I call the "windshield wipers." You lie on your back, bend your knees, and place your feet wide apart on the mat. Then, you allow your knees to drop to the left and right, back and forth like windshield wipers. I had cued the movement to match the breath: inhale the knees one way and exhale the knees the other way to slow the movement down and pay close attention to how it felt.

This young woman's knees were flopping from side to side without any control whatsoever. I went over to her and asked, "What would it feel like to slow this movement down like you're going in slow motion?" She looked at me with wide eyes and replied, "Umm, it's really hard." I said excitedly, "I know, it is hard! But with practice, it gets easier."

I figured I had sold her on the power of slow movement for bendy bodies. Unfortunately, she never came back to class. The idea that what's difficult for you is exactly what you need is a tough sell. But the truth is we don't get better at anything without a challenge. When we are willing to take on the challenge, benefits await.

For the bendy practitioner, using asana specifically for proprioceptive training has benefits that reach far beyond the yoga mat. For those who struggle with clumsiness or poor balance, improving proprioception can serve them in everyday life. Focusing on specific degrees of movement can be an interesting way to turn asana practice into an exercise in proprioception and motor control.

Let's use the cat and cow posture as an example—a posture in which you inhale to arch into a backbend and exhale to round into a forward bend. Most of us are accustomed to going as far as possible in both directions (100 percent of the available range) without stopping along the way.

To turn this into an exercise in proprioceptive awareness, I could move my spine only 25 percent of the way in both directions. After a couple of breaths like that, I might increase the amount of movement to 50 percent, and so on (See Figures 7d–7g). It requires focused attention to sense these various degrees of spinal movement and grade muscle contraction accordingly.

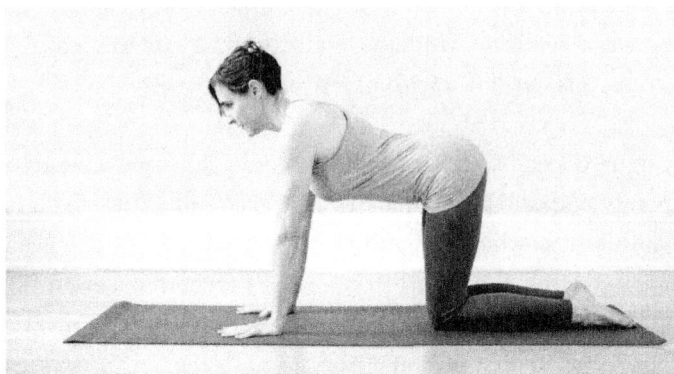

Figure 7d

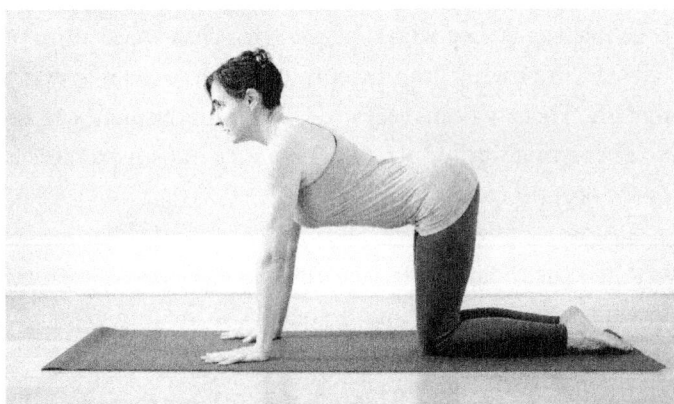

Figure 7e

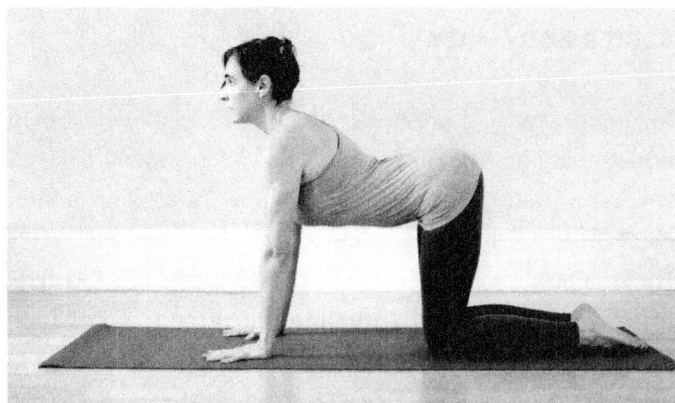

Figure 7f

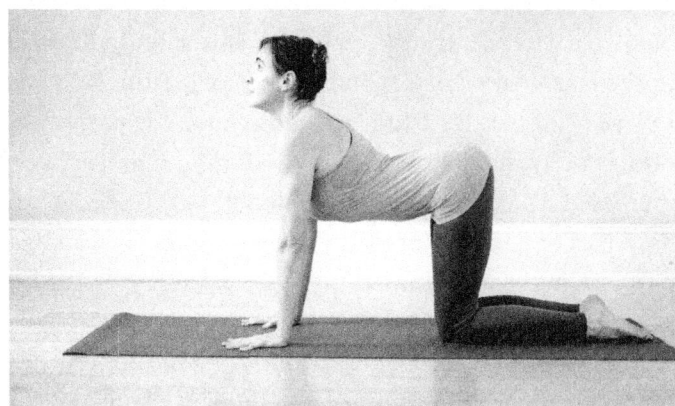

Figure 7g

When I do this, I can almost feel the connections between my brain and my body getting stronger. The same techniques can be applied to any dynamic asana or sequence of asanas. Again, in the beginning, many bendy practitioners will need external feedback to determine how far they've gone in each direction and to learn how it feels to be at each position along the way.

BETTER BODY MAPS

In the chapter "Common Bendy Body Complaints," I mentioned that bendy people's brains had been shown to have a smaller parietal cortex, which is where the somatosensory cortex is located. It's essentially the brain's map of the body. The smaller parietal cortex volume is thought to contribute to impaired proprioception, motor control, and coordination. The good news is that the brain is changeable.

One of the mechanisms by which the brain changes is in response to how we pay attention to and move our bodies. Movement helps shape and organize the brain. When we do an activity frequently, the real estate in the brain devoted to the task grows and becomes more well-defined. When I played competitive tennis in high school, the part of my brain's body map devoted to my swinging muscles likely increased. In contrast, when we don't pay attention to or use a part of the body for a long time, the brain's map of that part gets fuzzy and shrinks.

Slow movement is even better at clarifying the brain's body maps than moving at a faster pace. In his book *The Brain's Way of Healing*, psychiatrist Norman Doidge discusses the importance of slow movement for the brain's ability to clarify and differentiate its body maps. He states, "Slowness of movement is the key to awareness, and awareness is the key to learning.... Slower movement leads to more subtle observation and map differentiation, so that more change is possible" (Doidge 2015).

One of the reasons I love asana practice is that it consists of whole-body movements requiring attention to all our parts. Varying the specific way we practice asana requires we pay attention in new ways. And paying attention to our parts is what grows and refines our brain's map of those parts. As the body map gets more refined, our interpretation of sensation becomes more accurate, so our movements can be better controlled and coordinated. Research has shown that regular yoga practitioners increased the volume of their parietal cortices, among other brain benefits (Villemure et al. 2015).

Smaller and slower movements can be a portal to better proprioception, motor control, and body mapping for any practitioner. For the bendy practitioner, they are key to establishing boundaries, learning to put the brakes on movement, and developing a sense of containment. Many bendy people have shared that finding physical containment within asana practice helps them feel more grounded, connected, and integrated in other areas of life as well.

If you're a yoga teacher, I encourage you to invite your students to explore smaller and slower movements and get curious about what they discover in the in-between places. If you're a practitioner, see what happens when you approach your asana practice in this way as well. See what you've been missing in the gray zone.

CHAPTER 8:

Stretching

———

"If it's irritating, there's actually an easy fix:
stop doing it."

If there's one thing that gets people fired up about hypermobility, it's the question about whether stretching is good or
bad for bendy people. Should they stretch? Should they not?
What type of stretching is best? Many people are adamant
that stretching is terrible for bendy people. Others are equally
committed to the opposite view.

Stretching is complex for three main reasons. First, there's
a lot of misinformation out there about what we are doing
when we stretch. Yoga teachers and movement professionals
don't all have a unified understanding of what it means.

Second, there are many ways to stretch tissues. As I'll discuss below, we can stretch actively, passively, dynamically, or statically. Different types of stretching will likely produce different results.

Third, stretching is not only a mechanical event but also occurs in a human body where perceptions, thoughts, feelings, and our nervous system's assessment of threat always plays a role in our experience. In the body, nothing is purely mechanical.

In this chapter, I'll hit the highlights of stretching as it relates to hypermobility. Let's start with a description of what we generally think of as "stretching."

Stretching a muscle moves its attachment sites away from each other, thereby lengthening the muscle. The stretch places tension (a pulling force) on the tissue. In effect, stretching *is* tension. When I do a lunge with my left foot forward and my right foot back, the muscles on the front of my right hip and thigh spread out under tension, and I feel the tug (See Figure 8a).

TYPES OF STRETCHING

There are many ways to stretch tissues. The most common forms of stretching typically used in asana practice include dynamic, static, active, and passive. Dynamic stretching is when you move slowly into and out of a stretch repeatedly, such as you might find in a vinyasa style class. Dynamic stretching is usually active, meaning you use the force of your own muscles to create the movement into and out of the stretch. Of course, the more slowly you move, the more active your muscles must be to control the movement.

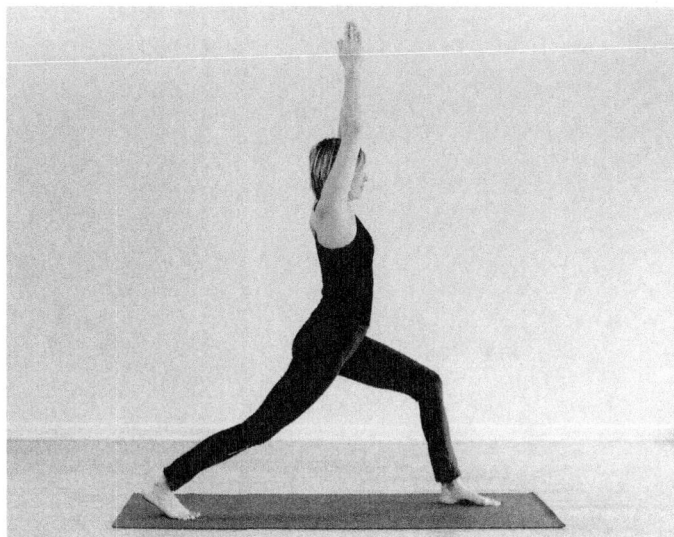

Figure 8a

Static stretching is where you hold a stretch for some amount of time. Static stretching can be performed passively by using an external force to hold you in the stretch position. The external force can come from a yoga strap, gravity, another body part exerting pressure, or another person. An example is using a yoga strap to hold your leg up in the reclining big toe pose so that your arms are doing the work and the leg is relaxed (See Figure 8b).

A passive stretch simply means I'm relaxed while in the stretch. It doesn't necessarily have to occur at my end range, but it could. For example, I could flop into the pigeon pose and passively hang out at my end range (See Figure 8c).

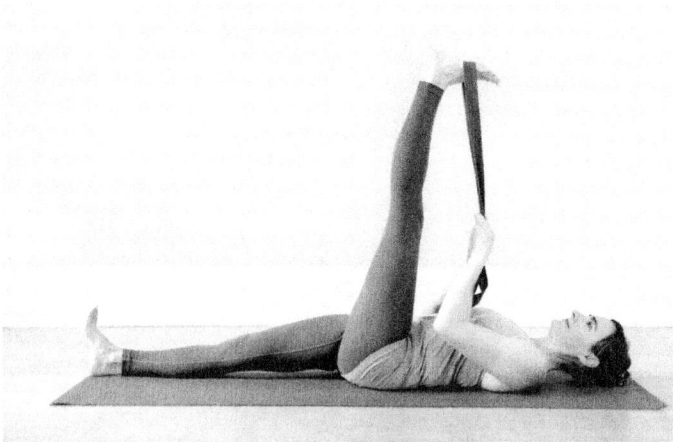

Figure 8b

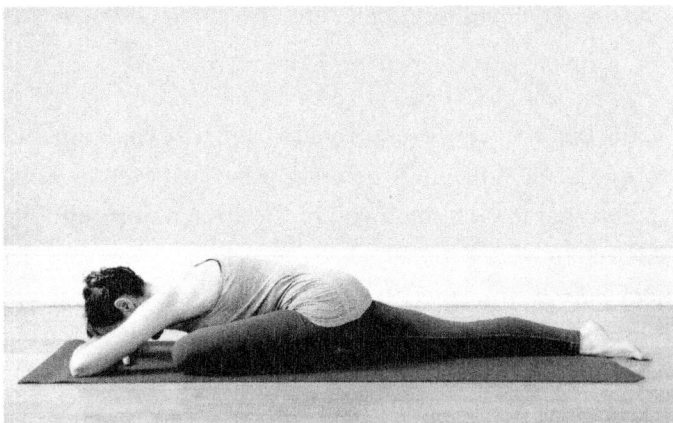

Figure 8c

Or I could relax into the pose with support underneath me so that I feel a less intense stretch and avoid going all the way to my end range (See Figure 8d).

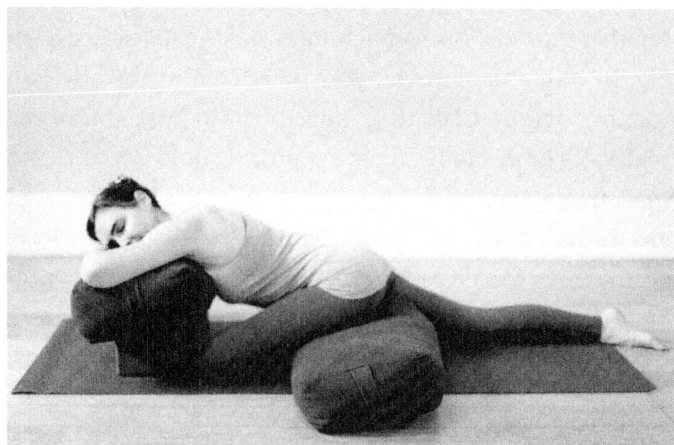

Figure 8d

Static stretching can also be performed actively by using your own muscles to hold the stretch position. An example would be using your muscles to actively hold your leg up toward the sky in a reclining big toe pose (See Figure 8e). In this case, I'm contracting the muscles in the front of my thigh to stretch the muscles in the back of the thigh.

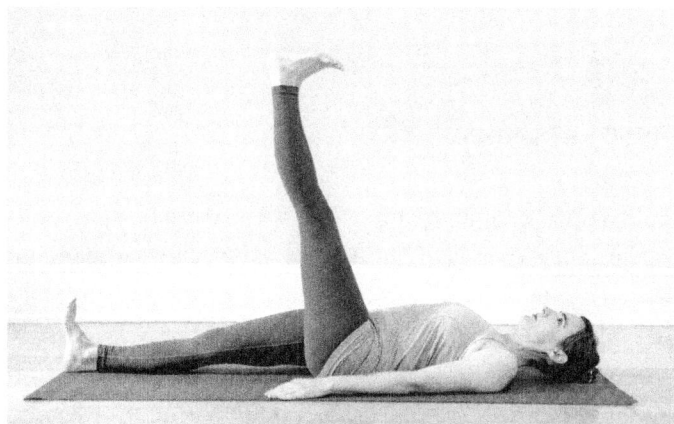

Figure 8e

Another type of active stretching is called isometric stretching, in which the muscles you are stretching are also contracting, without creating movement, to hold you in the position. For example, in pigeon pose, I could isometrically contract my leg muscles as if I were going to draw my knees toward each other (See Figure 8f). The active isometric form of stretching can be particularly beneficial for bendy people for reasons I'll discuss below.

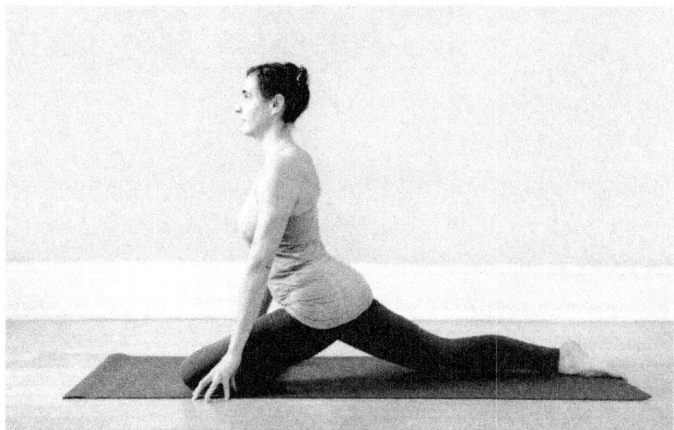

Figure 8f

TISSUE RESPONSE TO STRETCHING

Sometimes people mistakenly believe stretching actually makes muscles longer, but instead, it just spreads them out. When a muscle first senses a stretch, it contracts to resist it—this is a reflexive mechanism to prevent muscle injury in instances where the tensile load is too great. If the nervous system perceives the load as safe, it takes around twenty to thirty seconds for a muscle to relax and spread out to its full length.

After a stretch, a muscle returns to its original length fairly quickly. That's called an elastic response to stretching. Easy deformation; easy recoil.

Connective tissue responds differently and takes longer to respond to a stretch. When placed under tension for long enough—usually three to five minutes—it becomes softer and deforms (changes shape) by lengthening. Deformation of connective tissue is called "tissue creep." When you remove the stretch, it takes a longer time to recoil to its original length. This is called a viscoelastic response to stretching (Stecco 2015).

In the chapter "Connective Tissue Nitty-Gritty," we established that bendy people's connective tissue isn't as good at resisting stretch. It deforms more easily and recoils even more slowly than "standard issue" connective tissue. That means it creeps more and stays "creeped out" for longer (Stecco 2015).

We also established that tensile loading stimulates connective tissue to become stronger and better able to withstand the load, as described by Davis's Law. While all connective tissue, bendy or otherwise, is strong and resilient, it does have its limits. It is possible to stretch connective tissue to the point of damage, at which point it cannot recover its resting length. That is called a plastic (permanent) deformation and indicates tissue failure (Stecco 2015).

Animal studies have shown that unrecoverable damage to collagen fibers can occur following prolonged tensile loading. The damage has been observed even before tissue rupture and can result in permanent changes in tissue behavior such as even easier deformation and slower recoil (Zitnay and Weiss 2018).

More research is needed to fully understand human connective tissue response to stretching with various load parameters, such as frequency, duration, magnitude, and so on. It certainly would be helpful for our purposes if some of that research could be carried out on people with hypermobility syndromes. Specifically, I would like to see research that explores how tensile loads that lead to improved tissue strength differ from tensile loads that lead to damage.

WHICH STRETCHING IS BEST FOR BENDY PEOPLE?

Some well-meaning movement professionals and healthcare practitioners caution hypermobile people against stretching at all. I've certainly had people warn me about the grave dangers of stretching and direct me to strength training instead. While I agree with the bit about strength training (and I do it, albeit reluctantly), the bit about stretching is not so cut and dry.

In fact, while stretching and strength training generally have different intentions, they both apply a tensile load to your tissues. When you lift a barbell, your muscles contract and pull on their attachment sites; when you stretch muscles, the muscles lengthen and pull on their attachment sites. Despite these activities applying the same type of load to your tissues, the rate, magnitude, duration, and other load parameters vary widely. In particular, the magnitude (amount) of the load is greater during strength training (thanks to the presence of an external load) compared with stretching.

Stretching isn't inherently bad for bendy people, but prolonged passive stretching at end range can be problematic for many. Prolonged passive end-range stretching can lead to a longer period of decreased joint stability following the stretching session (Abboud and Descarreaux 2016). This is more likely to be a problem for bendy people because our floppy tissues don't recoil as quickly in the first place. Instead, they remain even floppier for a while after stretching. End range is also the place in the range of motion in which bendy people are most vulnerable to injury.

For many bendy people, end-range stretching of the hamstrings tends to be particularly irritating. Many practitioners develop hamstring tendinopathy—chronic hamstring tendinitis at its attachment to the sitting bone—due to excessive forward folding to end range. Some people refer to this as "yoga butt," and it's one of the most common complaints I hear from bendy yoga practitioners. For some, even if stretching their hamstrings feels good in the moment, they have more pain in the days following.

The reason passive end range stretching tends to be irritating for bendy people isn't well understood. Some research suggests the tendon irritation may be the result of lateral compression on the tendon as it presses into the sitting bone during a forward fold, rather than the tensile load of the stretch itself

(Docking et al. 2019). A lot of factors likely contribute, including the lateral compressive load, frequency and duration of the load, and the lack of other forms of loading that could improve the tendon's ability to withstand the passive stretch.

For example, research suggests that strength training can improve tendon stiffness even for bendy people, so the tendon is better able to withstand stress (Moller et al. 2014). It's possible that for many bendy people, the problem isn't as much "overstretching" as it is chronic underloading of the tissue. Active muscle contraction like the isometric stretching I mentioned above is one way to increase tensile loading during stretching and may yield more favorable outcomes.

Iryna Merideth is a bendy yoga practitioner and teacher in Carrboro, North Carolina. In a recent conversation I had with her, she shared this is the case for her. She has a delayed negative response to passive end range stretching but responds better when she resists the stretch through isometric muscle contraction. She explained:

> I don't always feel anything in a stretch, so I have to go really far into the pose to feel a lot of sensation. There's something satisfying about that in the moment, but I've learned it's not always the best idea. I've been working on accepting that I can't just jump into the stretch and allow gravity to take over. I have to apply a lot more muscular engagement. Otherwise, things hurt, especially after a really stretchy yoga class. Twenty-four hours later, I find myself wondering, "Why are my joints hurting?" It's like my body is saying, "No. Not so far. Not so deep."

For many bendy yoga practitioners, me included, reducing the frequency of passive end-range hamstring stretching, and importantly—adding resistance training to improve the tendon's capacity to withstand stress—helps a great deal. After years of resistance training, I don't have the same response to passive end-range hamstring stretching that I used to have.

First, my range of motion has changed, and my sensory awareness has improved. I can feel the sensation of stretch much sooner than I used to. Second, thanks to the resistance training, my hamstring tendons are stronger and aren't as irritated by longer duration stretches.

There's another reason adding resistance to a stretch can be helpful for bendy people. As I mentioned before, stretching is not only a mechanical event. It's also a sensory event, and we all perceive and interpret the sensation of stretch slightly differently. If you're a yoga teacher, you may have had students ask, "What is this supposed to feel like?" If you're a practitioner, you may have asked this question yourself.

It's difficult to answer because all of us don't experience things in the same way. Nonetheless, general guidelines about the qualities we are after when we stretch soft tissues can help.

I often describe it like this: "We're going for a mild-to-moderate sensation of tug, spread across a broad area of soft squishy tissue. It isn't sharp or pin-pointed at a joint or muscle attachment site; it's well-distributed." Stretch doesn't need to be extreme. In fact, the body often responds with more willingness to relax when the stretch is mild to moderate.

A big challenge for bendy people is that sometimes they don't feel anything in a stretch, especially in a passive stretch. They can go all the way to their end range and never catch that well-distributed sensation of tug across their tissues. They usually either feel a sharp sensation at a joint or muscle attachment site—or nothing at all.

In a recent conversation with Trina Altman, a yoga and pilates instructor with hypermobility, and the author of *Yoga Deconstructed®: Movement science principles for teaching*, she shared some of her early experiences of stretching in yoga classes and described how she was finally able to feel the sensation of stretch.

I could drape my elbows on the floor in a forward fold and feel no stretch in the backs of my legs. I'm so floppy, my joints just went everywhere. What really changed things for me was adding external load.

Like many bendy people, she needed some resistance to help her feel the sensation of stretch in her body. In yoga postures, resistance can be applied by pushing against something (such as a strap) or by contracting muscles to resist the stretch, such as in isometric stretching.

The active pigeon pose I mentioned above (See Figure 8f) is one example of an isometric stretch. Another example would be the big toe pose with a strap (See Figure 8b), but this time pressing my leg into the strap to resist the stretch. This type of stretching can provide the sensory stimulation bendy people often need to feel their bodies stretching.

In addition to the mechanical and sensory aspects of stretching, research suggests stretching may stimulate cells within connective tissue to release molecules called resolvins, which help resolve inflammation (Berrueta et al. 2016). Other research indicates stretching may play a role in tumor reduction (Berrueta et al. 2018). Still other research suggests regular stretching can lead to improved sleep and cultivate a calming effect on the nervous system (Inami et al. 2014; Montero-Marín et al. 2013; Tworoger et al. 2003).

Whether stretching is calming or agitating for a specific person depends on how their nervous system perceives it at that moment. For me, if I stay in the realm of "mild to moderate" and "well-distributed" sensation, I find stretching has a calming effect. However, if I force a stretch to my end range, it agitates my system. For example, if I let myself drop fully into the pigeon pose as far as I can go, it sets off my nervous system alarms (See Figure 8c).

However, if I support myself with bolsters or other props, then I feel a mild stretch that is quite nice, and I'm able to relax and enjoy the pose (See Figure 8d).

Iryna Merideth described a similar experience. When she got curious about the more subtle sensations of stretch arising before she reached her end range, she found a sense of safety she hadn't expected. As she explained:

> I started to do less, and by doing less I mean just backing out of the stretch by maybe 10 percent. And I started noticing that I was breathing more easily. And there was a subtle sense of safety. I realized when I

would go really deep into a posture, if I listened carefully, internally, I would notice there wasn't a feeling of safety. There was a feeling of competition and pushing. Now I've learned if I come out of the pose a little, I can still feel all sorts of other stuff. It's hard because it's such a paradigm shift to practice this way.

Through practice and much trial and error, Iryna has discovered an approach to stretching that works for her. It isn't irritating for her tissues and doesn't set off her nervous system alarms.

Clearly, stretching and our response to it are complex. If you have more discomfort after stretching, it's not an indication for more of the same. If it's irritating, there's actually an easy fix: stop doing it. You may need to try a different form of stretching, stay in a smaller range of motion, or add some resistance. In general, dynamic and active forms of stretching don't tend to be as irritating for bendy people but can still scratch the stretching itch. The best research you can do comes from experimenting with different types of stretching in your own body and studying your response with curiosity rather than expectation.

CHAPTER 9:

Strength and Stability

———

"Despite being able to deadlift 120 pounds
without much problem, I have a hard time
taking my arms all the way overhead from
a supine position without subluxating
my shoulders."

In nearly all conversations I have with people about hyper-mobility and yoga, the topic of strength and stability comes up. Although asana practice is not primarily a fitness pro-gram, many people come to asana with fitness goals. For bendy people, asana presents a great opportunity for improv-ing strength and stability.

Improving strength and stability is universally important for bendy people for several reasons. First, they've been shown to have decreased muscle strength and endurance (Coussens et al. 2021; Rombaut et al. 2012). Second, their muscular system is under even more demand for support due to the relative laxity of their passive connective tissues. Before we go any further, let's review the types of muscle contractions.

TYPES OF MUSCLE CONTRACTION

Muscles can contract in three different ways: concentric, eccentric, and isometric. Concentric muscle contraction is when a muscle shortens. When I bring a heavy water bottle to my mouth, I'm contracting my biceps brachii muscle to do the task, and it is shortening along the way.

Eccentric muscle contraction is when a muscle lengthens under a load while still contracting to resist or slow that load down. When I lower my heavy water bottle back down after taking a sip, my biceps brachii muscle still has to contract in order to slow the movement down. The muscle is contracting at the same time it lengthens.

Isometric contractions are when muscles hold you steady in a posture without moving. If I pause my water bottle halfway up to my mouth and hold it steady right there, my biceps brachii muscle is contracting to hold my arm steady, but no movement is happening at the joint.

An isometric contraction on both sides of a joint simultaneously is called a co-contraction. In my water bottle example, I'd hold my water bottle steady somewhere on the way to my mouth and imagine I was both bending and straightening my elbow at the same time. It wouldn't look any different than a simple isometric contraction, but it would feel different.

STRENGTH AND STABILITY

Strength and stability both have to do with muscle function, but they mean different things. Strength is the ability to create movement against some external force to get a task done. Strength would describe your ability to use your (generally larger) muscles to get yourself (or a kid or barbell) up off the floor using concentric and eccentric muscle contractions.

Stability is the ability to hold steady and to use your (generally smaller) muscles to resist unwanted movement during a task. Stability describes your ability to control joint position throughout a task through isometric or co-contractions.

If I'm doing a deadlift, I want to use the strength of my hamstrings and gluteus maximus to create movement at the hip joints. But I also want to use the muscles of my core to resist movement between the segments of the spine to ensure my trunk stays steady while I do the lift.

Strength and stability are both important for optimizing physical function. Plenty of bendy people can get a task done with their big muscles but ask them to fine-tune the control of their trunk or maintain joint stability during a task, and it's much more difficult.

While asana practice can provide opportunities for improving muscle strength, I think stability is where asana really shines. Yoga asanas are prime settings for cultivating muscular engagement to support joints and resist unwanted movement, as well as to fine-tune motor control for stability in motion. Core stability and joint stability are two relevant topics here.

CORE STABILITY

The "core" is an intriguing concept and is often misunderstood. When you hear the common verbal cue to "engage your core" during yoga class, the teacher often means to contract your abdominal muscles in some way. But the core describes a much broader area.

I like to think of the core as a box surrounding the abdominal cavity. The top of the box is the respiratory diaphragm; the bottom is the pelvic floor muscles. Around the front and sides of the box is the deepest abdominal muscle layer, transversus abdominis. Lastly, the back of the box is the deep lumbar multifidus muscle which provides segmental stability for the spine. An even more comprehensive concept of the core includes all of the trunk muscles in addition to the shoulder and pelvic girdles (shoulder and hip muscles).

When performing their stability function, the core muscles all work together as a team to resist motion in the center of the body when you're under a load. An example would be my ability to use the muscles in the center of my body to resist movement during a plank pose so I can hold the position.

Several common yoga asanas offer opportunities to cultivate stability in the trunk and pelvis, including plank, side plank (See Figure 9a), and tabletop balance, otherwise known as "bird dog" or "quadruped" balance (See Figure 9b).

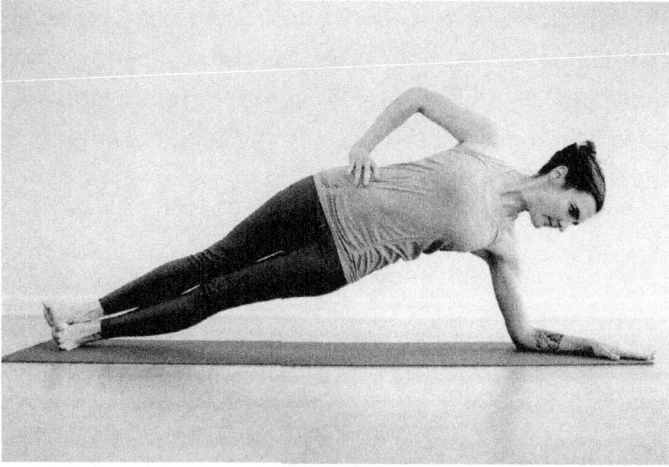

Figure 9a

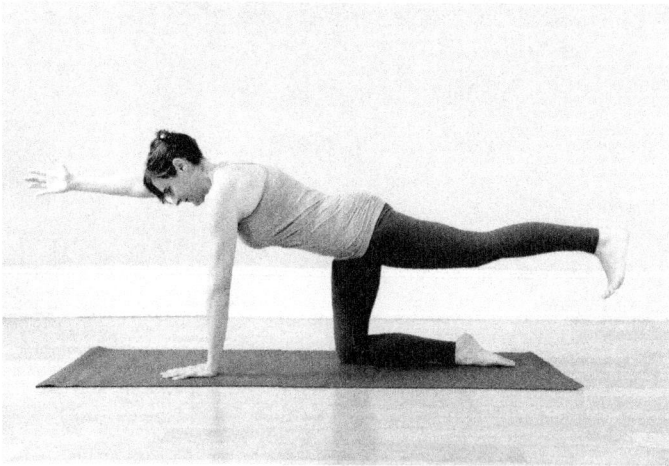

Figure 9b

Furthermore, I always recommend including postures that specifically target the muscles of the back and hips to support pelvic stability. This is particularly useful for people who struggle with sacroiliac joint pain. My favorite postures for this include bridge pose (See Figure 9c) and locust variations (See Figure 9d). In both cases, I encourage bendy practitioners to keep the posture lower to the ground—this can often help them focus on actively engaging the muscles in the back of the hips (gluteal muscles).

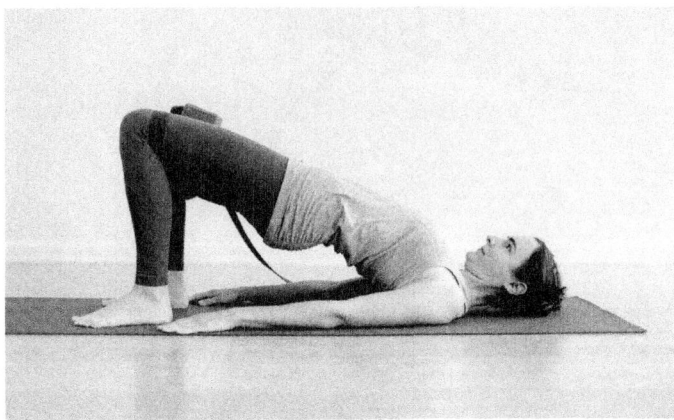

Figure 9c

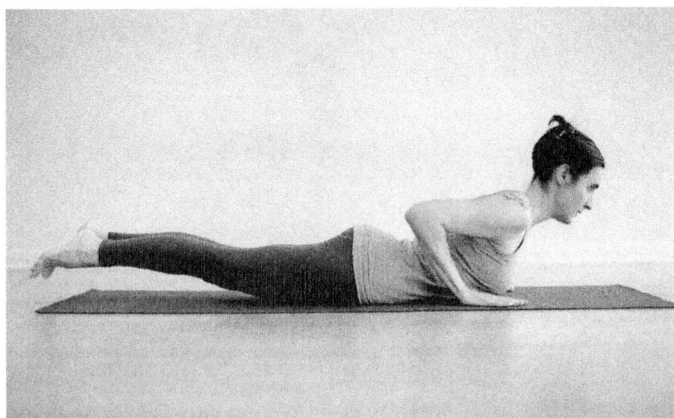

Figure 9d

JOINT STABILITY

For all bendy people, but especially those who dislocate or subluxate frequently, joint stability is the name of the game. Joint stability is being able to either maintain a joint's position or control its movement while maintaining joint approximation (the connection between the bones that form a joint).

Muscular contraction around a joint is the key to joint stability. When you consider all the various ways you could perform each yoga asana, you'll likely find opportunities to emphasize stability everywhere you look. In the chapter "Stretching," I discussed a few different ways to practice the pigeon pose.

To emphasize hip joint stability, I could do an active version. For example, I can keep my torso upright and draw my two knees toward each other isometrically (without any movement) to create a supportive muscular action in my legs and stabilize my hips (See Figure 9e).

To do it differently, I could allow my pelvis to sink as far as it can toward the floor and flop into a relaxed forward fold without any muscular contraction stabilizing my hip joints (See Figure 9f).

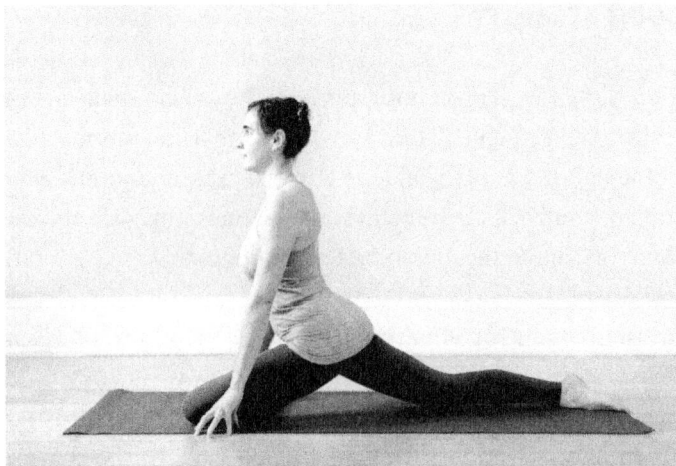

Figure 9e

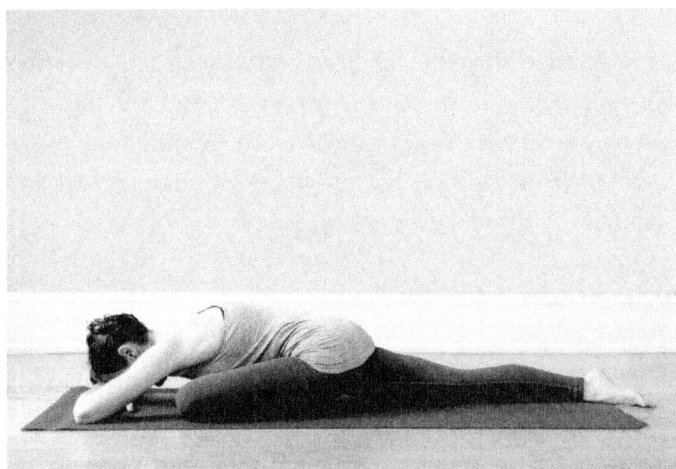

Figure 9f

These are very different pigeon poses. One is oriented toward stability (the active way), and the other is oriented toward mobility (the floppy passive way).

Maintaining joint position also relates to the common issue of elbow and knee hyperextension. A lot of bendy people hyperextend elbows or knees (or both), meaning they can straighten those joints so far they appear to bend backward. The reason for this is because their ligaments, some of which are designed to limit hyperextension, are floppy and don't do a good job restricting it. This reduced restriction can contribute to ligament sprains and decreased stability for the joint.

A common cue heard in yoga classes to address hyperextension is to "micro bend the joint," meaning bend the joint a tiny bit to avoid hyperextending. I often hear this cue in table top balance or plank pose to address hyperextending elbows and in triangle pose to address knees (See Figure 9g).

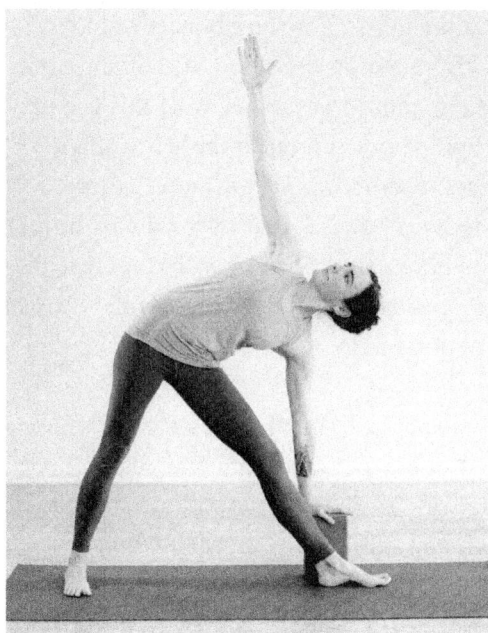

Figure 9g

Micro bending a joint can be helpful, especially when there's discomfort or significant instability at that joint. However, sometimes bendy people's joints flop into rotation when they micro bend them. For example, when I micro bend my front knee in the triangle pose, my thigh tends to flop into internal rotation, so my knee cap faces inward. Better muscular control of my micro-bent knee keeps it in a more comfortable and stable position.

A micro bend by itself won't necessarily help the muscles around a joint stabilize it. This is when co-contraction comes in handy as a better strategy to actively create joint stability (Hirokawa et al. 1991).

Co-contraction means to contract muscles on both sides of a joint simultaneously. For the elbow, it would feel like bending and straightening the elbow at the same time, without allowing any movement to occur. If this is a new concept for you, hold your arm out to the side and give it a try! In yoga classes, I sometimes hear the verbal cue to "hug your muscles to your bones." That's what a co-contraction feels like. If you have a static style of asana practice in which you hold each posture for some length of time, you can explore co-contraction in any active posture.

Suppose you have a dynamic asana style in which you move in and out of postures, or from one posture to the next in a flowing way. In that case, you have an opportunity to focus on maintaining joint approximation (the connection between the bones) during your practice. The key will be slowing down to improve proprioception and motor control, as I discussed in "Smaller and Slower Movements" (Riemann and Lephart 2002).

One of the things I have to focus on in my practice is shoulder joint approximation. Despite being able to deadlift 120 pounds without much problem, I have a hard time taking my arms all the way overhead from a supine position without subluxating my shoulders. This means when I lie on my back and take my arms up and back toward the wall behind me, I lose the connection between my humeral head and my glenoid fossa at some point (around 160 degrees) (See Figure 9h). My humeral head essentially pops out of the glenoid fossa, making a distinctive clunk.

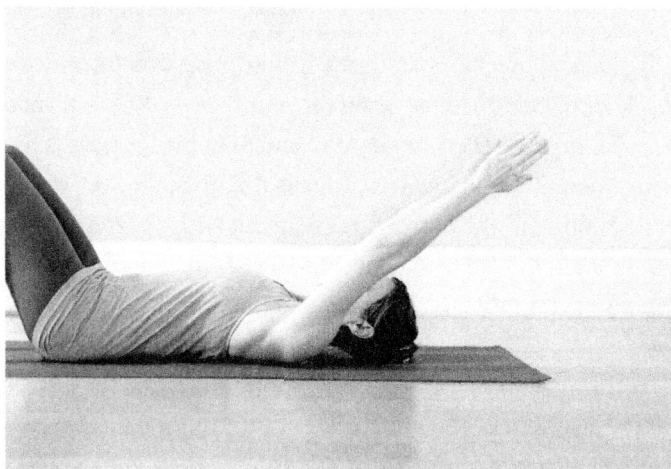

Figure 9h

To improve my joint stability in this movement, I have to slow down and use my shoulder muscles to control it only as far as I can without the humeral head popping out of the socket. It's hard work! As is the case for many bendy people, my available range of motion isn't the same as the range of motion I can actually control. My ability to control this movement has improved with continued practice and will likely continue to do so. Remember, controlling movement at midranges is the foundation for controlling movement at end ranges.

COMPENSATION STRATEGIES

One of the superpowers of bendy people is they are expert compensators, meaning they can make movements happen using dysfunctional patterns of muscle recruitment and contraction.

I'll give you an example. In the bridge pose, you lie on your back with your knees bent and lift your hips up off the ground (See Figure 9c). The primary movement in bridge pose is hip extension. The gluteus maximus is the prime mover of hip extension, and the hamstrings help out with the movement. As such, to do the bridge pose, we ought to use the gluteus maximus and the hamstrings.

A common compensatory pattern for hip extension is a lack of engagement of the gluteus maximus, often referred to as "gluteal amnesia" (McGill 2007). This is when your gluteus maximus is sleepy and doesn't contract as well as it could when you need it to; other muscles then have to compensate for its laziness. It's thought to reflect a poor neuromuscular pattern in which your brain has gotten into a habit of recruiting the wrong muscles, or muscles in the wrong order, to do the task (Gilpin et al. 2020).

When it comes to bridge pose, people with gluteal amnesia often report a lot of engagement in their hamstrings, so much so that they often cramp. They also often report discomfort in the lower back. That's because the hamstrings and the lumbar muscles (especially quadratus lumborum) will do all they can to extend your hips even while the gluteus maximus is snoring. The bridge pose won't necessarily look different on the outside, but it sure will feel different on the inside.

In some cases, a yoga teacher's verbal cues can actually contribute to poor neuromuscular patterns. For example, many yoga teachers have been taught to specifically cue their students not to use their gluteus maximus during the bridge pose and others that require hip extension. When we intentionally teach our body to use an impaired recruitment pattern, it can be even more difficult to break.

This points to a critical need for yoga teachers to develop anatomical and biomechanical proficiency. It's very difficult to speak competently about what's happening in the body without understanding it. If you are a yoga teacher, let this be a gentle nudge in the direction of more anatomy study.

When you understand what's happening in the body during specific movements, it can be helpful to guide students' attention to those areas. This can help students gain body awareness and ultimately transform their compensatory patterns.

Let's say I'm in bridge pose, and all I can feel are my hamstrings cramping. If you tell me I'm supposed to use my gluteus maximus, I'll have an "aha" moment. Now I can consciously ask my gluteus maximus muscle to contract when I do that movement and notice how it changes things.

To complicate things a bit, bendy people often have a hard time locating and contracting the proper muscle for a task—that's part of why they tend to have so many compensatory habits. For many, resistance helps stimulate the muscle to contract. In the example of bridge pose, pressing thighs into the resistance of a strap can help stimulate a contraction in the gluteal muscles so the practitioner can learn what the contraction feels like.

There remain all sorts of debates about the perils (or not) of gluteal amnesia when it comes to back pain, knee pain, and other complaints (Spinelli 2019). Nonetheless, improving awareness about habitual compensation strategies is useful for bendy people.

Kate Skinner, a physical therapist in Montana who specializes in treating people with hypermobility syndromes, describes the unique talents bendy people have when it comes to compensation:

> My hypermobile clients are master compensators. If they need to do something, they can come up with fifteen different ways to do it, and most normal people could never possibly do it that way. I had a client about ten years ago with knee issues. Her form looked great when she did her exercises, but it wasn't until I hooked her up to biofeedback that I realized she was not using her quadricep muscles at all while doing squats or sit to stand. She was doing everything with

her medial hamstrings! So, you can't necessarily just watch somebody to know what's going on when they're hypermobile. They need to know, "This is where you should feel it."

I used to experience this myself in the chair pose, which is a squat of sorts. I had struggled with chronic sacroiliac joint and hip pain, and I was working on building my hip and leg strength. My brain had a hard time recruiting my gluteus maximus and medius (the outer hip muscles) during the pose, which allowed my knees to fall inward (See Figure 9i). For many months of practicing, I never felt those muscles engage; instead, I felt discomfort in my low back and knees. My body was trying with all its might to do the task using an impaired recruitment pattern.

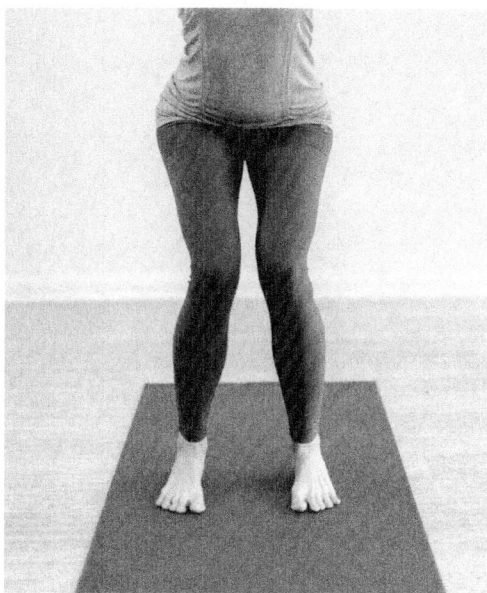

Figure 9i

Changing the pattern wasn't easy to do. I had to focus intently on using my gluteal muscles in this posture. Like many, my body needed resistance to figure out how to contract those muscles. Pressing my thighs out into a strap helped me learn what it feels like to engage those muscles for more stability (and more comfort) in the pose (See Figure 9j). Eventually, I learned to contract them even without the resistance of the strap. Even better, my chronic sacroiliac joint and hip pain began to melt away.

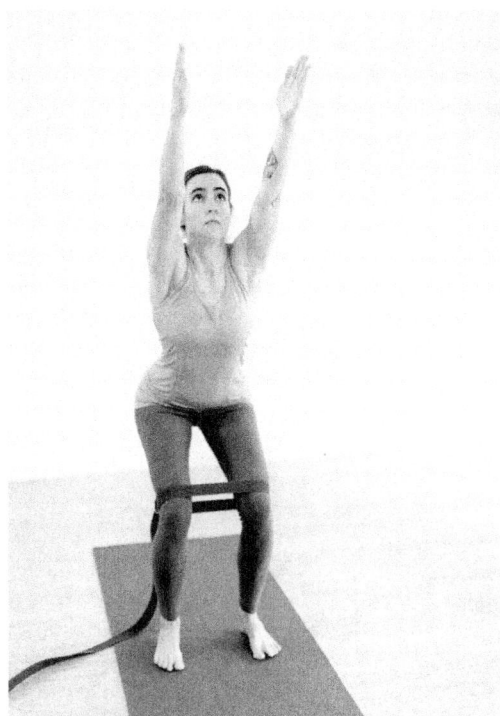

Figure 9j

The key to overcoming dysfunctional compensation patterns is slowing down so you can pay close attention to what's happening in your body. It's also helpful to learn which muscles should contract to perform a certain movement. Once you learn more functional recruitment patterns, you can bring that awareness into your yoga asana practice for better results.

If you're a bendy person, I encourage you to pursue some form of strength and stability training, even if it means signing up with a personal trainer who's knowledgeable about hypermobility syndromes. When it comes to yoga practice, it will likely serve you to incorporate some of the core and joint stability strategies discussed in this chapter. Asana offers a rich opportunity for stability training that is functionally relevant to living life in a bendy body.

CHAPTER 10:

Posture

———

"Posture is complicated, but the main cue
I give for it is simple: 'Back it up and
stack it up.'"

Posture is a slippery word. Most of us have been told all our
lives to sit up straight and beware of the perils of poor posture. But what does posture even mean? And more importantly, what *is* good posture?

Posture is the way our body parts stack up when we are
upright in gravity. There isn't much consistency out there
about what "good posture" means, although yoga teachers
and practitioners tend to place a lot of value on it. You've
probably heard yoga teachers dole out rote postural cues
in yoga classes, especially in tadasana, or mountain pose.
Those of us who are yoga teachers have undoubtedly done
the doling.

THE PROBLEM WITH POSTURAL CUES

Common standing posture cues used in yoga classes include "lift your chest," "pull your shoulders back," "tuck your tailbone," or my personal favorite, "lift your kneecaps." You may have also been told to "equally weight the four corners of your feet" or "internally rotate your thighs."

Each of these cues leads to a change in the position of the body. In order to know whether those changes are desirable, I need to know what the "good posture" goal is. Otherwise, I cannot cue my yoga students in the direction of said good posture.

As if that wasn't challenging enough, we don't all start out in the same place. Yoga practitioners with different postural features will need different cues to reach the good posture goal—if it does indeed exist.

For example, in any given yoga class, some students' pelves (that's plural for pelvis) are probably posteriorly tilted with the tailbone tucked under, and some are anteriorly tilted with the tailbone sticking out behind them. Still, others are probably somewhere in between. So, what cue should I give my class about what to do with their pelves? It's tricky.

As much as I'd love to blame everyone's back and neck pain on their unsavory posture, available evidence doesn't show a convincingly strong correlation between the two for the general population. For example, some research shows low back pain isn't related to the amount of curve someone has in their lower back (Laird et al. 2016). Other research shows that people without back pain slouch just as much as the rest of us (Claus et al. 2016).

On the other hand, I see bendy patients all the time who feel better when they gain awareness of their habits and adjust their posture. I certainly know that my posture impacts my pain and fatigue daily.

Research suggests that people with hypermobility syndromes display different postural habits than their non-bendy counterparts and have a more difficult time maintaining upright positions (Booshanam et al. 2011; Bates et al. 2021). They also demonstrate differences in muscle activation patterns during standing and decreased proprioceptive sense of their position (Rigoldi et al. 2013; Greenwood et al. 2011).

When it comes to whether or not posture matters, the issue seems to be twofold. 1. Posture may not matter as much as we wish it did for the general population, and 2. Posture matters more for bendy people than others.

WHY POSTURE MATTERS FOR BENDY PEOPLE

I recently had a conversation with Dr. Lilian Holm, a physical therapist in Illinois who specializes in treating people with hypermobility syndromes. We talked about the particular relevance of posture for bendy people, given their unique qualities.

The question is not whether posture matters in general. I think the question is, "When does it start to matter for a particular person?" For someone with a hyper-mobility syndrome, there's probably a way to relate to gravity that is better, more comfortable, and more easeful. It's about our body's adaptation to imposed demands. In a hypermobile population, you're dealing with tissue that's very different. There's decreased stabilization from inert structures, which allows us to go a little too far in various directions, applying forces to tissue that by definition is weaker. The only conceivable way of compensating for that would be to rely more heavily on stabilizing muscles.

It's common for hypermobile people to fatigue easily when in an upright position. That's why you'll often see them leaning on furniture, walls, or any other external support. Without solid support from floppy connective tissue, the muscles of bendy people have to pick up the slack, which means they work extra hard. It's tiring and can also lead to muscle tension and pain.

In a recent conversation with Jill Miller, yoga therapist and author of *The Roll Model*, she illustrated the effect of forward head posture on the upper trapezius (the muscle on either side of your upper back and neck) as an example. When you hang your head forward like we often do at our computer and other devices, she described your head like a big tuna fish hanging on the end of a fishing pole.

The fishing pole has to strain and bend and elongate faster on the top of the fishing pole than it is on the bottom. The strain impacts the entire back of your body, but it puts greater stress on the upper trapezius muscles that are trying to reel back that tuna, or reel back that head. The only way a muscle knows how to reel it back in, is to contract. So, the muscle stays in a chronically contracted state to help bring your head back over your body.

Some bodies can tolerate more of these postural habits than others, and the bendy body is likely to be one that responds with more pain and irritation to them.

Aside from the imbalance of passive versus active postural support, decreased proprioception (sense of joint position and body awareness) also contributes to why posture matters for bendy people. When people have a hard time accurately sensing where their body is, it's harder to notice the habits that lead to discomfort. It's also harder to sense when the body is in a more optimal position.

Kate Skinner is another physical therapist in Montana who specializes in treating hypermobility syndromes. In a recent conversation I had with her, she reflected on the impact impaired proprioception has on posture for bendy people— particularly bendy yoga practitioners. She explained:

> The thing that is most surprising to people is they feel like they have really good posture because they work really hard on it — particularly the yoga instructors. It's never an effort issue. They're working so hard they kind of miss the mark.

She describes a strong postural habit in her bendy yoga-practicing patients in which they lift their chest and retract their shoulder blades excessively, creating a swayback appearance. This common habit puts their shoulders in a position where they can't work as effectively, leading to weakness and other upstream problems for the neck.

The harder they try, the worse it gets because they don't realize where a normal thoracic curve actually is. When you put them there, they feel like you're making them slump. They feel like, "Oh that's terrible posture!" And I have to stick them in front of a mirror, and I have to show them. I think it speaks to the fact that so often, we're not the best objective measures of ourselves when there's hypermobility.

Getting accurate feedback about where the body is in space is one of the greatest challenges for hypermobile yoga practitioners. They often work so hard that they just blow past the target because it's so difficult to sense those places of postural integrity from the inside out. External feedback such as a mirror can help bendy people learn what it feels like to be at their target position. With practice over time, they can learn to find that position without relying on the external feedback.

Kate's story about her yoga-practicing patients is consistent with an interesting study on children with hypermobility. When they were given an external postural cue to "straighten your back," they tended to overshoot their target and end up in a similar swayback position (Czaprowski et al. 2017). The researchers concluded that giving a hypermobile child that type of postural cue simply wasn't effective due to their proprioceptive deficits.

In my recent conversation with her, Lilian Holm echoed the importance of proprioceptive training for posture. She emphasized that being at an end range is how many bendy people are able to feel anything at all and understand where their body is. Sitting or standing doesn't generally place our joints at end range unless we flop significantly, so it's much harder to discern where we are. As she explained:

> A lot of people with hypermobility habitually lean into end range positions because activating the mechano-receptors and feeling where the body is, feels very good. It is actually very important to our experience as human beings to be able to orient ourselves in this time space reality and know where our boundary ends and the rest of the world begins.
>
> It's a question of learning. What does our nervous system learn to rely upon? If hanging out at end ranges is the only way you know where your joints are in space, you will not be as good at picking up the subtle signals of being in a neutral position. With training, people can learn to sense where their body is without having to go to extreme end ranges, but it's a gradual process.

There are some things we can explore to make posture more efficient and comfortable for bendy people while supporting improved proprioception at the same time. Happily, they are also things well suited for incorporating into a yoga asana practice.

Posture is complicated, but the main cue I give for it is simple: "Back it up and stack it up."

BACK IT UP

Learning to back it up and stack it up is one of the most important and difficult things I've ever tried to do with my body, but it has made a big difference.

Many bendy people tend to drift their pelvis forward so it lines up over their toes rather than over their heels (See Figure 10a). "Backing it up" means to do a simple but mindful weight shift so that the body's center of mass (the pelvis) rests over the heel bones instead.

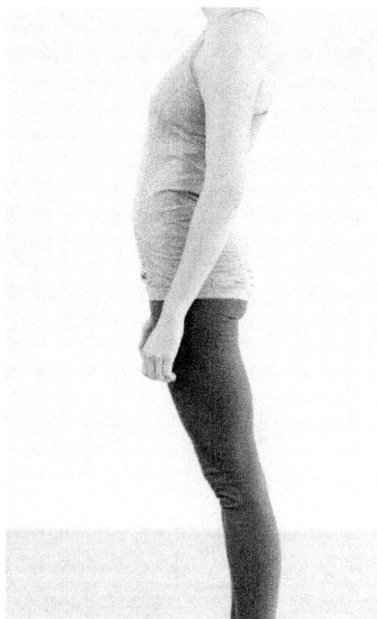

Figure 10a

Backing up the pelvis also changes its tilt, allowing it to find its way to a neutral-ish position. Neutral-ish is a highly nontechnical term to describe a position that approximates neutral, or "middle of the road." What's a neutral-ish pelvis? I'll give you my take on it, learned from one of my favorite voices in biomechanics and the author of several excellent books, Katy Bowman.

Bowman describes establishing a neutral pelvis by lining up the ASIS (Anterior Superior Iliac Spine) with the pubic bone vertically when you're standing (Bowman 2014). The ASIS is the front pointiest part of the big bone on either side of your pelvis that forms the "shelf" where you rest your hands sassy-style on your hips. Your pubic bone is in the front of your pelvis down low, forming a bony shelf at the very bottom of your low belly. You can also explore this lying down on your back by tilting your pelvis forward and back until those bony landmarks line up horizontally with each other.

Our bones are all shaped slightly differently, and that can make it difficult to get an accurate assessment of pelvic position (Preece et al. 2008). I'd rather encourage people to go for neutral-ish instead of getting carried away with a ruler. Feeling the position of our bones with our hands is not an exact science, but it's a useful starting point.

STACK IT UP

When we back up the pelvis so the center of mass lands over the heel bones, we have more weight in the heels than the forefeet. Then, our bones begin to stack up on one another: The shin bone stacks on the heel bone, then the thigh bone stacks on the shin, and finally, the pelvis stacks on the thigh bone.

From the pelvis, we can keep stacking by inviting the ribcage to stack over the pelvis. If the pelvis is a bowl, the ribcage becomes its lid. For the rib thrusters out there who tend to throw their low ribs forward into a swayback, that means dropping your front lower ribs to restore a natural (rather than excessive) lumbar curve.

Lastly, reach the crown of your head toward the sky without jutting your front ribs forward into a back bend (See Figure 10b). This is especially important for people with kyphosis, or excessive thoracic curve. Extending the spine by pressing the crown of the head upward isn't meant to completely flatten out the spine; it's meant to decrease excessive forward rounding of the thoracic spine and get the head back over the rest of the spine instead of hanging forward.

This sounds complicated (and it kind of is), but I have a few tips that can help.

First, I like to lightly place a yoga strap around the lower rib cage—which is another tip I got from Katy Bowman (go read her books) (Bowman 2016). The strap allows you to sense the position of your ribcage. If you tend to flare your front ribs forward, it can help you bring some awareness into the back ribs instead. Once you sense the position of your rib cage, you can begin to breathe into the full circumference of your rib cage, so it spreads out in all directions and makes contact with the strap.

For a little help figuring out what it means to press the crown of your head up toward the sky, I like to use a head cushion developed by Esther Gokhale, author of *8 Steps to a Pain-Free*

Back (Gokhale 2008). A standard eye pillow will also do the trick. Place the head cushion or eye pillow right on top of your head so that when you press your head up into it, the back of your neck lengthens a bit (See Figure 10b). Try this standing or place your back against a wall for support.

Pressing your head into the cushion stimulates the muscles along your spine whose job it is to hold you upright. When they discover how to hold your upper back more upright, the whole upper body takes on a different shape. The shoulders often fall into place even without the cue to "squeeze your shoulder blades together."

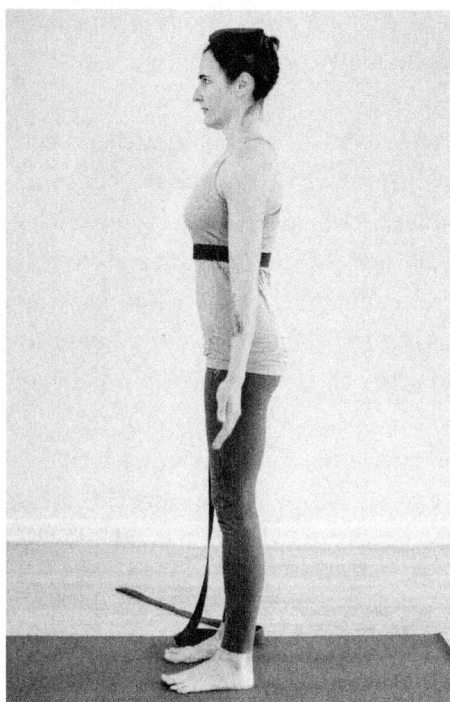

Figure 10b

The strap and the head cushion give the body feedback about where it is in space. After some practice with this, you'll have an easier time finding your way to a more neutral-ish posture on your own. Mindful practice will help your nervous system learn to pick up the cues of a more neutral position, and you may even be able to replicate the feeling of it within other asanas in your practice.

Maintaining prolonged upright positions is usually not comfortable for bendy people. They prefer to keep moving. Ideally, when we learn to stack our body parts in a neutral position with natural spinal curves restored, our bones can support our weight without so much muscular effort. Then, holding ourselves upright for longer periods of time is less fatiguing and, hopefully, more comfortable.

Whether you're a practitioner or a teacher, I encourage you to go on a postural adventure and try out some of the tips in this chapter. Get to know the relationship between your pelvis and rib cage. Discover how it feels to restore the natural curves of your spine. Explore how shifting the weight in your feet changes the rest of your body upstream. Use a mirror and other external feedback to help you. Find out how changes in postural habits can impact your breathing, fatigue, and muscle tension, to name a few. Worry less about perfecting a certain shape and be more curious about feeling your way into a new way of dealing with gravity.

CHAPTER 11:

Designing an Asana Practice

"When you give your body more of what it wants and less of what it doesn't want, you get good results."

So far in Part Two, we have discussed several key considerations for optimizing asana practice for people with hypermobility syndromes, including smaller and slower movements, stretching, stability, and posture. In this chapter, I'll outline a few additional things to keep in mind, such as sequencing, movement variety, positioning, dose, and frequency. Finally, I'll discuss a few asana precautions.

SEQUENCING

Designing an asana sequence is complex. First, you have to choose which postures you want to practice. Then, you must decide how you want to practice them—dynamically, statically, and with this or that variation. Finally, you must place those postures in a specific order or sequence. That's a lot of moving parts!

Sequencing is about linking postures together such that the practice cultivates positive effects while minimizing negative effects (Desikachar 1999). Sequencing is a complex art and science worthy of an entire book, but I want to focus on a few key elements I find most relevant for bendy people.

In some popular styles of asana, there seems to be a game going on in which the instructor creates a sequence of ten to fifteen different postures on one side of the body and then wows the class with her ability to remember the entire sequence on the other side. That's an example of a highly asymmetrical sequence.

While long asymmetrical sequences can be a fun challenge, it is also likely to exacerbate musculoskeletal pain, leaving bendy practitioners feeling wonky after class. Wonky is a highly non-technical term I use to mean generally unhappy, tweaky, or otherwise out of whack.

So, what is an asymmetrical posture? Asymmetrical postures require you to perform both sides. For example, you do triangle pose on one side and then the other side. Symmetrical postures are just done once. Chair pose is a good example of a symmetrical posture. For bendy people, asymmetrical postures aren't inherently problematic, but they become so when many of them are strung together in a row.

I used to frequent a fairly vigorous hot flow yoga class taught by a friend of mine a couple of times per week at my home studio. I love this friend's teaching because she does such a good job weaving yoga philosophy into her classes. However, the asana sequencing is usually a bit faster and less symmetrical than my body likes.

Because I already knew I needed more symmetry, I made modifications throughout the practice. I moved a bit slower than the others, limited my range of motion to about 75 percent, and inserted rogue symmetrical postures frequently throughout the class. If I did these things, I came out feeling great.

A few years ago, I did an experiment. I thought to myself, "You know, you've been doing a lot of strength training over the past decade, and your body is stronger than it's ever been. I think you could handle doing this class full-throttle. Why not give it a shot?" And I replied to myself, "Sure, why not?" So, I did the class without my usual modifications for two weeks. I moved with more momentum, went to my end range, and didn't bother inserting my usual symmetrical postures along the way.

By the end of those two weeks (a measly four classes), my low back was hurting in an old familiar way that I hadn't experienced in a long while. And the alignment of my pelvis was noticeably out of whack. Bodies with hypermobility tend toward pelvic asymmetries, meaning the two sides of the pelvis aren't even with each other. One side could be elevated or rotated forward or back, or the whole thing could be rotated to the left or right.

While some bendy bodies have consistent asymmetries, others will keep you guessing. Things move around more in a bendy body. One day the left side of the pelvis is elevated; the next day, the right side is elevated and rotated forward. It's okay to be asymmetrical; in fact, most bodies are. But for a bendy body, it's more common for asymmetries to be problematic and to be exacerbated by highly asymmetrical asana sequences.

I told my teacher friend about my experiment and its results after class one day. She stepped back to look at my body and said, "Wow, I can totally see your pelvis is all rotated and wonky. That's crazy!" Happily, everything got back on track quickly once I resumed my usual modifications.

The moral of the story: once a bendy person, always a bendy person. If I want to enjoy my friend's hot flow yoga class, I will always need to make those modifications because they are what make that style of asana practice work for me. The same is likely true for many other bendy practitioners as well. Those modifications served to compensate for the potential ill effects of the practice.

Many teachers are familiar with the concept of compensation (sometimes called the "counterpose"), accomplished by following each posture with one that brings the body back to balance, so no ill effects are carried into the rest of the practice. For example, a gentle forward bend would be the counterpose for a backbend (Desikachar 1999).

Adequate compensation throughout an asana practice is important to optimize the benefits for any practitioner. For people prone to aches and pains following practice, such as bendy people, it's even more critical. Consider symmetry to be the counterpose for asymmetry. More symmetry can minimize the ill effects of a practice while optimizing its benefits for bendy practitioners.

You can think about symmetry like the volume dial on your car stereo. You can turn it up or down according to how your body responds to the varying degrees. On the highly asymmetrical end of the dial, you'll do a long string of fifteen postures on one side. On the other end of the dial, you'll do one asymmetrical posture on both sides and follow it with a symmetrical posture.

There are two ways to infuse an asana sequence with more symmetry. First, include more symmetrical postures to give the body a chance to feel balanced. Second, limit the number of asymmetrical postures you perform at a time. Instead of ten (or more) asymmetrical postures in a row, do fewer. To find the right number for you, play around with this concept and see what your body tells you. I generally don't practice or teach more than two or three asymmetrical postures in a row.

MOVEMENT VARIETY

Next time you enjoy an asana class, take note of the variety of movement types being performed during class. For example, how many forward bends are included as compared to backbends, side bends, and twists? In some popular asana styles out there, you may perform fifty to sixty forward bends during a practice but only one or two back bends, and perhaps zero active backbends that focus on back strengthening.

For some reason, modern asana practice has become profoundly forward fold-centric, and this can be problematic for bendy practitioners. Deep forward folds to end range, especially when held passively in a relaxed way and done very frequently, tend to exacerbate the chronic sacroiliac joint pain and hamstring strain so many bendies experience.

In the chapter "What is Yoga?" I told you a bit about my decade-long struggle with these issues and how my (reluctant) willingness to stop excessive forward folding was key to my recovery. Bringing more movement variety into your asana practice can change everything. When you give your body more of what it wants and less of what it doesn't want, you get good results.

If you liked the volume knob analogy for symmetry, think of balancing your movement variety just as you would balance the sound to the four speakers of your car stereo. Instead of blaring the music from just one speaker (forward folds) and keeping the other three speakers silent (back bends, side bends, and twists), see what happens when you spread the music out a bit.

Movement variety is great, but there's also plenty of variety to be found *within* each asana. We tend to always perform postures the same way, especially if we've been taught there's only one right way to do each one.

In my practice and teaching, I generally do a similar set of simple asanas during each practice, but I vary how I do them. Tired of the same old bridge pose? How about placing your feet together, or wider apart, or making it a single leg bridge? How about pressing your arms into the floor, or lifting one or both arms overhead as you bridge? How about squeezing a block between your thighs, or pressing your thighs out into a strap? (See Figure 11a)

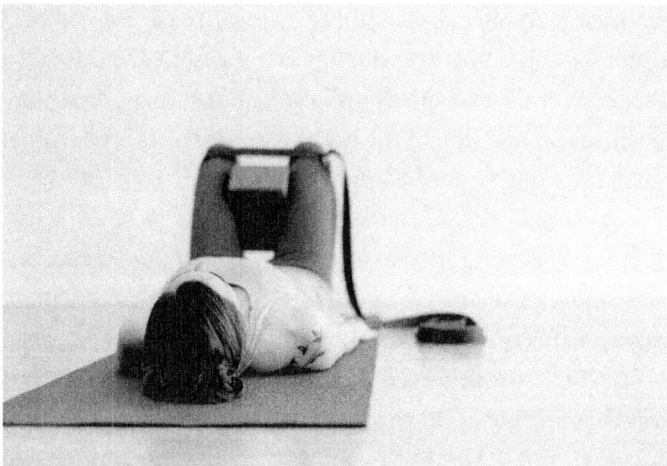

Figure 11a

Get creative, and you'll find there are seemingly endless ways to perform each asana. Our bodies and brains love variety and novelty. Doing new movements, and doing the same old movements in new ways, are powerful tools to stimulate growth and clarity in your brain's body maps.

FATIGUE

Fatigue is a common struggle for people with hypermobility syndromes. It can play a role in exercise tolerance and recovery, or it can be an obstacle to exercise at all.

During exercise, bendy people tend to become fatigued more quickly, in part due to decreased muscle strength and endurance (Coussens et al. 2021). Accordingly, they may benefit from more frequent opportunities for rest, or decreased hold times for static postures during asana practice. Aside from the other problems with asymmetry, performing ten or more postures on one side of the body is exhausting, especially if we're talking about standing postures.

I remember being in a yoga class in which the teacher led us through a seemingly endless string of standing balancing postures on one side. About halfway through, I looked around the room to see if anyone else seemed like they wanted to throw in the towel. I gave myself a few moments of support from my other leg, but since everybody else seemed happy, I carried on. By the end of the sequence, my standing leg was consumed by aching fatigue. It was barely able to support me at all. I still remember the sweet relief I felt when it was over.

Muscle fatigue isn't a bad thing. A bit of fatigue is required for muscles to get stronger. But too much of a good thing is usually a bad thing. If we keep pushing and pushing after our muscles fatigue, the body has no choice but to default to compensatory patterns in order to get the task done. If the right muscle for the job is exhausted, then other muscles have to step in to pick up the slack. Those compensatory patterns can lead to other problems.

Sometimes, general fatigue can be an obstacle preventing people with hypermobility syndromes from initiating or continuing a yoga asana practice. In the case of Chronic Fatigue Syndrome, asana practice may be significantly limited. Some days, yoga looks like lying in your bed, moving your arms and legs, and doing some basic breathing practices.

While physical activity can be a helpful component to recovery, it's important to find the type and amount of activity that doesn't leave you even more depleted. Sometimes that requires the assistance of a qualified healthcare provider.

Fatigue is also likely to impact someone who struggles with insomnia. Limiting stimulants and screen time in the evening, eating an earlier dinner, and using the bedroom purely for sleep (or other bed-specific activities) can be helpful. Making some adjustments to your asana practice is also wise. For example, I recommend doing more vigorous asana practices earlier in the day and emphasizing gentler calming practices before bed.

Because so many bendy people struggle with impaired exercise tolerance, adjusting the dose and frequency of asana practice can also be helpful. For example, instead of a seventy-five-minute practice, a twenty- to thirty-minute practice might work better. Instead of practicing six days per week, practice every other day. Instead of a vigorous class, try a gentler class sometimes. These are just examples. Everyone has to find their own unique parameters. At its best, physical activity leads to improved energy, not depletion.

POSITIONING AND HEAT

In the chapter "Common Bendy Body Complaints," I discussed the high prevalence of POTS (Postural Orthostatic Tachycardia Syndrome) and Orthostatic Intolerance (difficulty being upright) among bendy people. Someone struggling with these challenges would be wise to consider positioning. Emphasizing kneeling, prone and supine postures, or modifying standing postures to be performed kneeling or lying down, could all be good ideas. Simply offering the opportunity to change positions can be helpful.

Transitions between postures can be tough as well. A lot of ups and downs and abrupt transitions can exacerbate dizziness for people with POTS. On days my POTS symptoms are strongest (I call these "potsy" days), I spend more time close to the ground in yoga practice, lying on my back, my belly, or kneeling. To help with POTS symptoms, many people also benefit from compression socks, even during yoga practice.

Heat often compounds the struggles for both potsy practitioners and people with Mast Cell Activation Disorder (MCAD). Steering practitioners with these issues toward a non-heated yoga class is wise. Heat increases potsy people's risk of fainting and increases the chance someone with MCAD will leave class covered in hives.

For some people struggling with the symptoms of POTS, increasing salt or electrolyte intake can help keep blood pressure and heart rates in optimal ranges and reduce symptoms during exercise. As always, consult your doctor before starting any new diet or supplements.

ASANA PRECAUTIONS

As I discussed in the chapter "Common Bendy Body Complaints," a relatively high prevalence of craniocervical instability exists among bendy people. That means the joints where the neck meets the head are unstable due to ligament laxity. This predisposes people to Chiari Malformation and can cause more serious complications.

Because of these risks, I would urge caution with shoulder stand and headstand in practitioners who have a hypermobility syndrome. Without significant modifications, these postures place demands on the craniocervical junction that may cause more harm than good. When in doubt, consult your doctor or physical therapist about these risks.

I also mentioned bendy people's higher risk for shoulder dislocation because it's an inherently mobile joint (like a ball on a plate). It's wise to avoid placing the shoulder in the position of shoulder dislocation during asana practice, especially if it's weight-bearing. The most common position for shoulder dislocation is abduction out to the side with external rotation.

One yoga posture that makes me cringe because it puts the shoulder in exactly this position is the "wild thing." To get there, you start in downward dog pose, and then as some say, you "flip your dog" by lifting one leg (See Figure 11d), coming onto one hand, and turning over into a one-armed back bend (See Figure 11e). For most people, it's not a big deal. But for bendy people, I would steer clear.

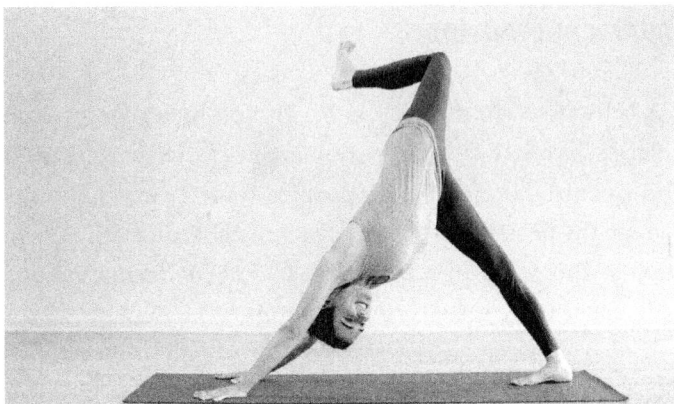

Figure 11b

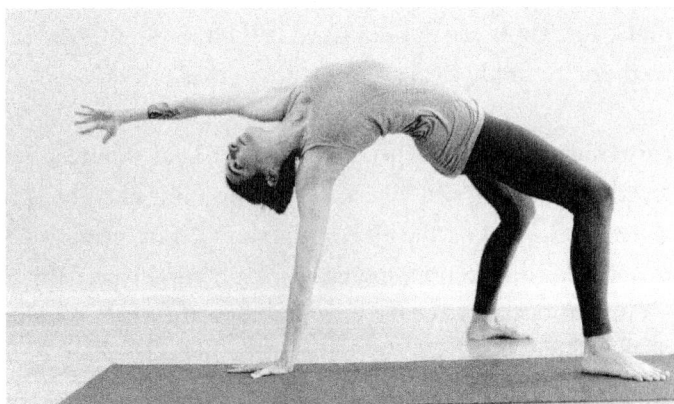

Figure 11c

Watch out for other postures that place the shoulder in a similar position. Even in the side plank, it's important to avoid pointing the head of the humerus forward. Instead, actively press your hand or forearm into the floor and hug your shoulder blade onto your back (See Figure 11d). Where shoulder instability is a concern, I would also avoid deep binding. "Binding" means wrapping your arms around yourself to clasp your hands together while you're in a yoga posture (See Figure 11e).

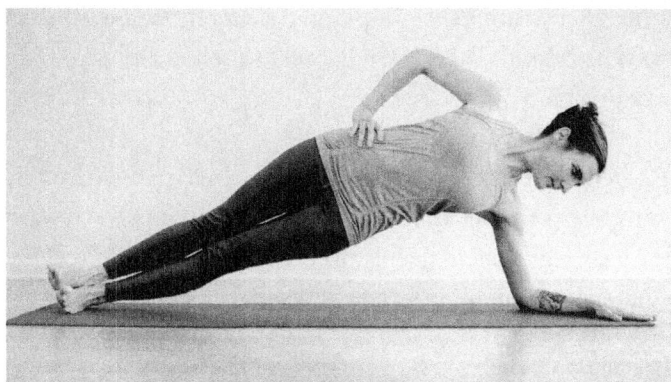

Figure 11d

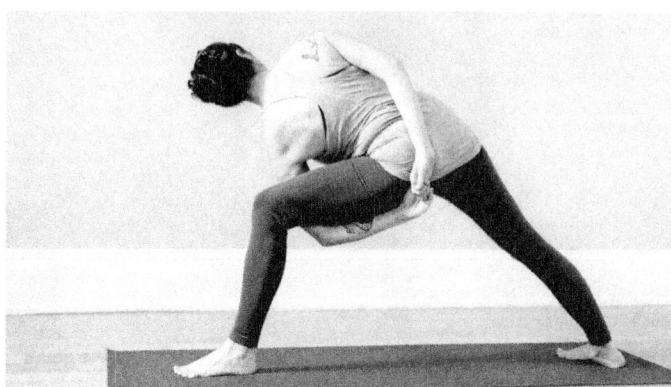

Figure 11e

Sacroiliac joint pain is the number one complaint I hear about from bendy yoga practitioners. It's characterized by a sharpish pain at the top of the sacrum where it meets the ilium, usually on one side or the other. Triangle pose, twists, and excessive forward folding tend to exacerbate it.

Many bendy people with sacroiliac joint pain have a love/hate relationship with triangle pose. They love it because when they're in the pose, they can really "feel it" in their sacroiliac joint. They assume the pin-pointed sharp sensation they feel must be helpful. They hate it because they seem to have more nagging pain afterward.

The version of triangle pose that seems to flare up sacroiliac joint pain is the one in which you swing your hips out toward the back leg and fold deeply over the front leg while keeping your spine straight, with feet wide apart (See Figure 11f).

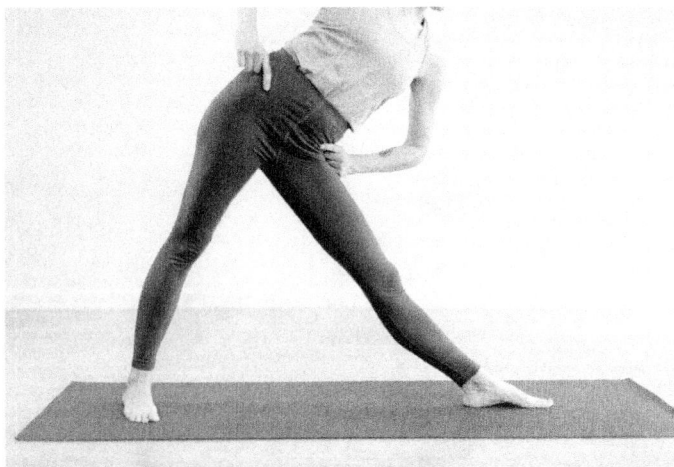

Figure 11f

Instead, I recommend narrowing the stance, keeping the pelvis stable (rather than doing the hip swing), and allowing the spine to bend sideways into the posture. Most people won't go nearly as far into the pose, so a block or chair under your hand can be helpful (See Figure 11g).

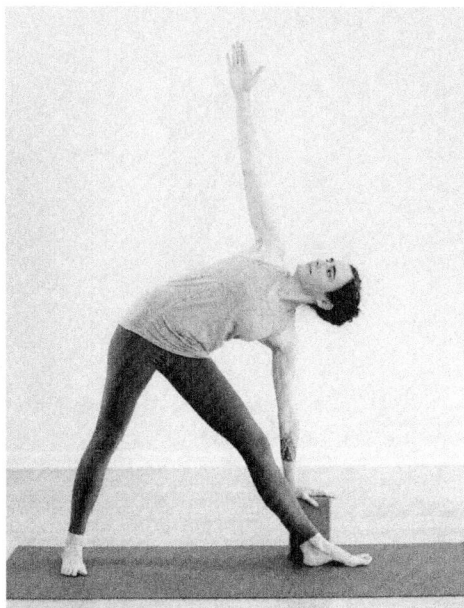

Figure 11g

Twists can also exacerbate sacroiliac joint pain, especially seated twists. In many seated twists, the pelvis is stuck to the ground, and the spine rotates on top of the pelvis. Things tend to be more comfortable when the pelvis is free to move into the twist a bit along with the spine. This is easier to do in supine twists. In general, I recommend people allow the pelvis some freedom to move in twists so that it's comfortable, instead of keeping it locked down in a certain position.

Excessive and prolonged forward folding is another common irritant for sacroiliac joint pain. Again, many bendy people assume they should do more forward folds because they really "feel it" in those postures. And again, many find they have more pain afterward (See Figure 11h).

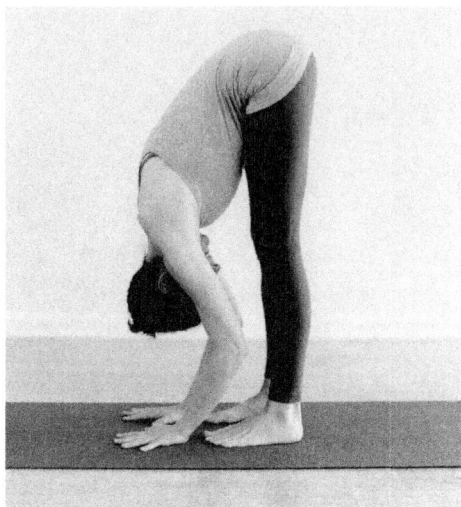

Figure 11h

As I discussed in the chapter "Stretching," excessive forward folding can also exacerbate the chronic hamstring strain so many bendy people struggle with. It tends to improve when they reduce or avoid passive end range hamstring stretching—at least temporarily—and supplement their asana practice with strength training.

Strengthening the muscles around the sacroiliac joint (your butt and low back muscles) with postures such as bridge and locust pose can be helpful (See Figures 11i and 11j). In fact, unless they are irritating, I recommend these postures be done daily. It's also helpful to bring more symmetry into your asana sequence, as discussed at the beginning of this chapter.

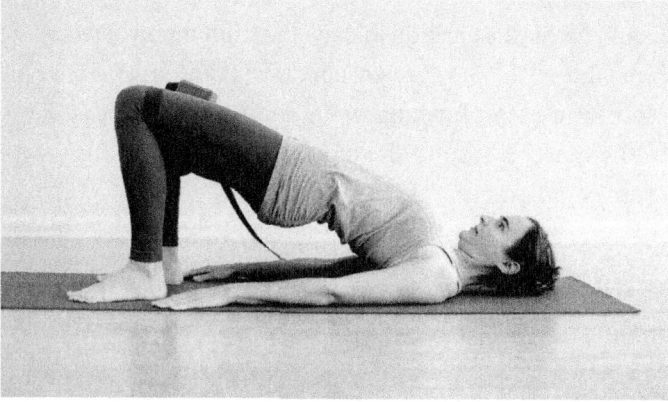

Figure 11i

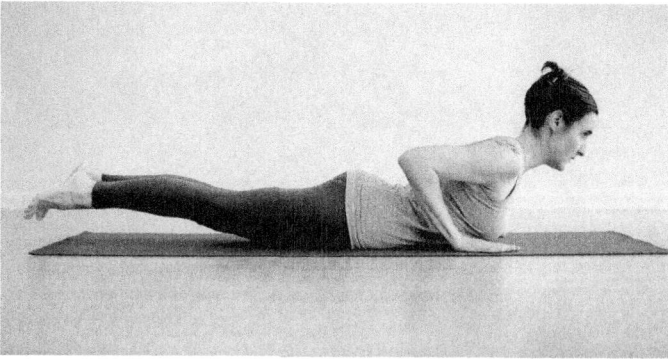

Figure 11j

Lastly, postures some refer to as "hip openers," which place the hip in some combination of flexion, external rotation, and abduction, often exacerbate hip pain for bendy yoga practitioners. This is especially true if they struggle with femoroacetabular impingement (when the hip labrum gets pinched between the femur and the hip socket) or a hip labral tear.

Examples of this position include the front hip in pigeon pose (See Figure 11k) and triangle pose (See Figure 11g). Generally, reducing extreme hip ranges of motion and building strength in the muscles around the hip can help tremendously with these complaints.

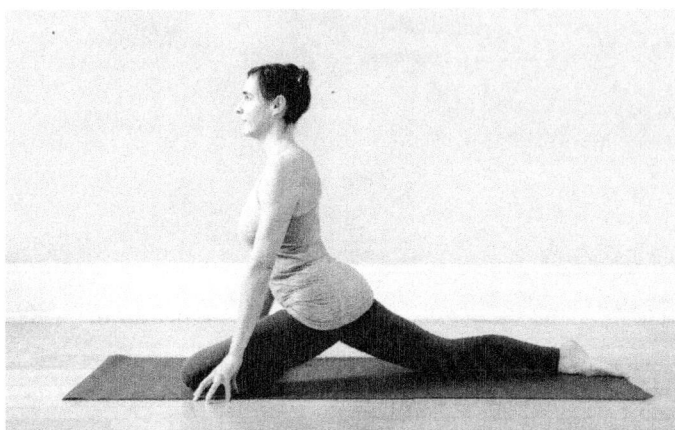

Figure 11k

I hope this chapter has given you some ideas about how to design an asana practice to optimize its benefits for bendy practitioners. Whether you're a teacher or practitioner, I encourage you to explore symmetry, movement variety, and positioning as you plan your practice routines. Balancing the dials on these aspects of sequencing can truly change everything for bendy yoga practitioners, especially if they usually feel wonky following asana practice.

Permitting yourself to modify aspects of practice such as dose, frequency, and temperature may also make a big difference. It's also okay to eliminate problematic postures altogether.

The specific asana precautions I've suggested here can serve as a starting point. Other postures may certainly be problematic for specific practitioners, and some I've mentioned won't necessarily be problematic for all bendy people. I've listed the most common ones I hear about and work with on a regular basis. Let these recommendations fuel your own investigation.

CHAPTER 12:

Language and Verbal Cues

———

"Before you know it, my awareness has landed smack dab in my body in the present moment. Well done, yoga teacher!"

Whether you're a yoga teacher or practitioner, you already know the importance of the language and verbal cues used in class. A teacher's choice of words communicates everything to students. They describe how to get into postures and how far to go. They relay safety concerns and indicate the relative value of one version of a posture versus another. I've worked with countless yoga teachers who report anxiety about verbal cues. They want to be sure they say the "right things" about each posture. Likewise, most yoga students probably assume their teacher is saying the "right things" too.

Most yoga teachers are taught a few basic cues for each posture in their teacher training and then pick up more ideas from other teachers. Over time, teachers develop a repertoire of verbal cues and teaching language that works for them. As teachers, it's easy to get into a habit of saying the same things over and over without examining *why* we say those things. But, if we don't examine our verbal cues and teaching language, we don't know if we're saying what we mean to say. For our bendy students, some of our habits may not be so helpful.

DESCRIPTION VS. CORRECTNESS

Most verbal cues begin as descriptors that help students understand the shape of a pose. For example, "Place the soles of your feet together and bend forward" would help guide students into the seated bound angle pose. Common verbal cues for Warrior I include, "Step one foot forward and bend your knee so that it's over your ankle. Then take your arms overhead."

Descriptive cues are helpful. They are critical for beginning students because they give them needed guidance and direction about the posture at hand. But they can get mixed up with notions about correctness, implying that doing the posture in some other way would be incorrect.

It's a big leap to go from description on one hand to correctness on the other hand. In the case of Warrior I, is there really an *incorrect* way to step one foot forward and bend your knee? There may be more comfortable ways to do the posture depending on who's practicing it. But correctness is a stretch.

From correctness, it's a slippery slope to safety. In yoga class, students are often led to believe that not only is this the correct way to do the posture, but doing it in any other way would be unsafe.

Back to our Warrior I example. If I bend my front knee so that it goes beyond my ankle (instead of just over my ankle, as the teacher told me), is it unsafe? I've heard plenty of yoga teachers say to bend the knee *just* over the ankle in order to protect the knee. Protect the knee from what? I'm not sure.

I recommend a little experiment. Next time you go up or down a flight of stairs (or get up off your toilet), watch what your knees do. You'll find bending your knees past your ankles is a completely normal and functional thing for human knees to do. Will some knees protest? Sure, and some knees don't like stairs (or toilets). But that doesn't mean bending your knees past your ankles is inherently unsafe.

It's difficult to break habits of performing postures in the way we've been taught is correct or safe, even when it doesn't feel right. Assuming there is one correct way to perform each yoga posture is problematic because we all have slightly different bodies with different needs. There's no reason to assume we should all perform yoga postures in the exact same way. This is a particularly sticky trap for many bendy yoga practitioners who work hard to get things "right" but, despite their rightness, keep having trouble.

Something that might surprise you: In my clinical experience treating injured yoga practitioners and teachers over the years, not a single one of them was injured because they were performing yoga asanas *incorrectly*. However, many were injured because they were performing asanas the way they were taught was correct. It just wasn't correct for their particular body. Alternatively, many were practicing asanas their body didn't want them to be doing, regardless of correctness.

An example of this is chaturanga dandasana, the four-limbed staff pose. This is a pose in which you begin in a plank position and lower yourself toward the floor while keeping your elbows in by your ribcage. Many teachers are adamant about the "correct" way to do chaturanga, but a lot of people develop shoulder pain trying to do this asana with their hands and elbows in the prescribed position.

I don't think chaturanga is an inherently *wrong* way to lower oneself to the floor, but out of all the possible ways, I do think it's a difficult one. Many people lack the upper body strength to do it without eventual pain and injury. In the absence of adequate strength, it quickly becomes fatiguing, and fatigue may lead to compensatory patterns. My shoulders might be able to handle a handful of chaturangas in a practice, but fifty? That's a different ballgame.

I'm not sure who decided this was the *right* way to lower oneself to the ground. I'm not convinced my Paleolithic counterpart would have pushed herself up over a rock ledge or lowered herself to the ground in the chaturanga position, and I doubt her friends would have chastised her about it, "Ahem…elbows!"

This is one asana I find many practitioners strangely committed to, regardless of their shoulder pain. One time, in a workshop for yoga teachers, I was discussing alternative ways to perform chaturanga. When I demonstrated a way to lower myself to the floor with a different hand position, I noticed one of the attendees looking at me with shock and dismay. She said, "But that isn't correct alignment, and it's not safe for your shoulders!"

When I asked her to explain why the alternate hand position made the movement unsafe for my shoulders, she didn't have an answer for me. I always encourage yoga teachers to investigate the *why* of their cues. Why is this way better or safer? Why is the other way unsafe? If you're going to say it in yoga class, you should have a good reason why.

Unfortunately, many yoga teachers don't have a solid enough foundation in anatomy and biomechanics to really understand the verbal cues they were taught to use. They simply get into a habit of using cues someone told them were correct without ever examining the *why* behind them.

Trina Altman, a bendy yoga and Pilates teacher and author of *Yoga Deconstructed®: Movement science principles for teaching*, shared a story with me in a recent conversation we had that illustrates this. She told me about a yoga class she used to attend with a teacher who had been trained in a particular alignment-based style of asana.

> One day in class the teacher was saying something like, "Inner spiral your shins," or "Take your shins in and thighs out." I remember afterward wondering, "What if somebody has tibial torsion, and their shins are already 'in?' Why would they go more 'in?'" So, I

asked her why we were doing that. And she said, "I honestly don't know. That's just what my teacher said is one of the universal principles of alignment."

One of the most important things I learned during my month-long immersion of yoga study at the Krishnamacharya Yoga Mandiram (KYM) was the relationship between the *how* and the *why* of yoga asana.

Asana isn't about correctness; it's about the person who is practicing. We all have different bodies, goals, and needs, and those differences impact how we should practice. A claim about "rightness" should always be followed by "rightness *for whom?*"

Many scenes from my time at the KYM are etched into my memory. Here's one of them.

Early in our immersion, we were practicing Warrior II in our daily asana class when a student asked the teacher, "How exactly should my back foot be pointing in this posture?" I looked to the teacher, eager for his answer, and saw a confused look fall over his face. It seemed he had no idea how to answer the question.

After some thought, the teacher asked, "Does your foot hurt?" The student shook his head no. Then the teacher made an almost imperceptible shrug of his shoulders and said, "Then you can put it in whatever position is comfortable."

If you'd been a fly on the wall, you could probably hear the gears grinding in our minds at that moment. The room was full of similarly-trained yoga practitioners, primarily from the United States and Europe. Most of us had arrived with ideas about *the correct way* to practice yoga postures, but not much idea about *why* those ways were correct (or even why we would practice them in the first place).

Instead of asking about "the correct angle" of the foot in a given pose, more useful questions to ask include, "Why am I doing this posture? What do I want out of it? How does it make the most sense to do the posture given my goals and the needs of my body?" Answering these questions will lead to the appropriate verbal cues. In other words, shifting our attention from form to function and from performance to inquiry is a step in the right direction.

FEAR-BASED LANGUAGE

When practitioners or teachers become attached to ideas about correctness in asana, it's a slippery slope to ideas about safety. From there, it's easy to default to fear-based language. This is often called "nocebic" language (nocebo is the opposite of placebo) because it carries with it an expectation of a negative outcome. Nocebic language generally reflects a fragility mindset about the body.

Some people consider the human body as an inherently fragile thing that breaks easily and requires great carefulness to move safely. Others see it as an essentially resilient thing that's adaptable, designed for movement, and able to respond to and grow from challenges.

If I bring a fragility mindset into class, my teaching language will reflect that. I may be more apt to use fear-based language such as, "Be really careful with this movement!" If someone reports some discomfort, I might respond by saying, "Oh my god, I'm so sorry. Did I hurt you?" Without intending, this type of language sends a message to students that their bodies are fragile and what they're doing in yoga class is inherently dangerous.

If I wanted to communicate some of the same intentions but use language that reflects a resilience mindset, I might say instead, "Pay attention as you move through this posture and notice the sensations that arise." In response to discomfort, I could say, "Tell me more about what you are feeling. What happens if you try it this way instead? Remember, you're always free to come out of a posture at any time."

The way we speak to and about students' bodies conveys a powerful message that may help form their own self-concept. Do I want students to see themselves as essentially fragile or essentially resilient? While I certainly don't want students to be uncomfortable during class, the way I respond to their discomfort is important. I can respond to it in a way that suggests it's very scary, or I can respond with curiosity and encourage exploration about how to relieve the discomfort.

One of my personal mottos is, "Normal human movement is not inherently unsafe." These bodies are designed to move, but paying attention is useful. When we encounter discomfort in asana practice, we can modify or skip the offending posture. If someone is concerned about their physical discomfort, they should be encouraged to have it evaluated by their doctor or physical therapist.

DEGREE OF MOVEMENT

While some verbal cues relate to the specific shape of a posture, others indicate how far to go in the posture. You may be told to "reach through your fingertips," or "find your edge," where "edge" means the place where you feel some sensation of stretch or the place beyond which your body can't go any farther. After you've been in the pose for a while, you may be encouraged to "find your next edge," that is, to sink even deeper into the pose.

When it comes to hypermobile practitioners, cues that encourage students to go as far as possible into a posture aren't helpful. Not only that, but in some cases, such cues may lead them to more pain and injury. Bendy people must learn to translate common cues differently for themselves.

Kate Skinner, a physical therapist in Montana who specializes in treating people with hypermobility syndromes, emphasizes:

> It's really hard to ignore a cue. It's hard to tell yourself, "Just don't do that." So instead, I tell people to add on to the cue mentally. If someone is saying, "Reach as far as you can through your fingers," then I just tell people to add on a section that goes, "Except for me because I need to stay here," or something that allows you to be an exception. You create a new cue that puts a stop

to the movement for yourself, so it doesn't just keep going endlessly. I also often tell my clients to stay out of that last ten percent of their range. That way, you stay more connected in your body, and you're trying less to reach out of it.

Bendy practitioners don't usually get anywhere useful when they're encouraged to keep going as far as possible. Sarah Blunkosky is a bendy yoga teacher in Fredericksburg, Virginia. In a recent conversation, she shared how difficult the process of hearing cues differently has been for her.

I really have no proprioceptive awareness of my own limits, especially in back bending. I love back bends, but I have no awareness of how far I should go because my body doesn't stop me on its own. I've been trying hard to limit myself in backbends like cobra pose; because when I go as deep as I can, even though it feels good in the moment, my back hurts for a couple days afterward. It took me a long time and a lot of pain and injury to be able to be in a class listening to the cues and recognize, "Oh, that's not good cueing for my body."

If you're a teacher and you use language that encourages students to go as far as possible into each posture, your invitation is to reflect again on the *why*. Why do you think it's better to go farther? I would argue there's usually not a good reason.

LINEAR LANGUAGE

Another problematic feature of some teaching language is something I'll call "linear language" because it implies there's somewhere we are trying to get to in each posture, and the closer we get to that end goal, the better.

Many teachers will demonstrate a variety of versions of a particular posture for their students. It's wonderful to give students options, but how the options are described matters. I've often heard teachers present posture variations like this: "For level one, try this. For level two, try this. And for the full expression of the pose, try this." Meanwhile, their demonstrations are becoming progressively more challenging.

Many people are led to believe that with enough practice over enough time, they might be able to achieve the "full expression" of a posture, usually meaning the most physically demanding or "stretchiest" version. I can tell you from personal experience that achieving the "full expression" of a yoga posture does not lead to a happier life.

Another version of linear language goes something like this: "For a beginner variation, try this. For an intermediate variation, try this. And for the advanced version, try this." It's a rare human being who wouldn't feel a sense of failure for being unable to do the advanced version of a posture. This language indicates there's something better about being more flexible or physically agile and that your performance of postures indicates how good you are at yoga. But we must remember that the goals of yoga have nothing to do with how you do postures or even *if* you do postures.

If you're a teacher in the habit of correctness, linear language, and go-as-far-as-you-can cues, it can be hard to know what else there is. Instead of linear language, I encourage teachers to present posture variations as tools to find different sensations or get different effects out of the posture. For example, if you do the triangle pose with your hand on a block versus without a block, you'll get a different effect. A high lunge with your hands on the ground feels different from a high lunge with your arms overhead. While the variations are all different, they have equal value as far as yoga is concerned.

Yoga teachers need to give students a place to start and guide them on how to do the postures. But the "right thing" to say about a posture depends on why you're doing it. What effect are you hoping to cultivate with a posture? Cue the posture in a way that cultivates the effect you're after. Your words will guide students' attention in that direction.

CUES FOR CURIOSITY AND INNER AWARENESS

I'm a big fan of using verbal cues to guide students' attention to various aspects of their experience and invite inquiry during practice. Rather than naming their experience for them, I try to invite curiosity about it. For example, instead of saying, "Feel how grounded you are," or "Feel how connected you are to the earth," I might say, "Notice the way your feet feel on the ground," or "Notice the sensation of your feet making contact with the floor."

This type of cue invites the student to be curious about how that sensation feels to them and the effect it has on their experience. Whether or not they feel "groundedness and connection," they are exploring how they feel for themselves, and that tiny shift can be quite empowering.

Asking questions during class is another method for directing students' attention inward. For example, after performing a pose on one side of the body, I might ask, "What can you notice about the sensations in the two sides of your body after that posture?" I'll also throw in something like, "There's no right or wrong way to feel," just so students understand this is only an inquiry. You can't get it wrong.

Another way to cultivate awareness is taking moments of pause between postures and using those pauses specifically for inquiry into inner sensation. I like to invite students to take a "noticing pause" from time to time during practice simply to tune in and feel their bodies and breath.

As I mentioned in the chapter "Smaller and Slower Movements," exploring varying degrees of movement can also help students cultivate inner awareness. My general approach is to encourage bendy students to stop when they get to about 80 percent of their available range of motion in any given posture. This ballpark figure helps them begin to gauge the amount of movement they're doing and to start pulling away from their end ranges.

Because it's so tough for many bendy people to sense the position of their body accurately, it's hard to know when they've reached 80 percent. Just to get their bearings, it can be helpful to go to end range and then back out of the position a little bit. Sometimes I'll cue people to "go to the edge, and then back away from the edge." Mirrors can also be extremely useful for this.

Melanie Downey is a bendy yoga and meditation teacher and longtime practitioner in Massachusetts. In a recent conversation with me, she shared her "80 percent" strategy for helping bendy students in her classes begin to sense inner sensation differently.

It's impossible to know what someone else is feeling. For me, the most important thing about teaching asana is to help people develop inner awareness, so they learn how they feel and learn what's working for them. I usually suggest that people with hypermobility go to 80 percent of their maximum range of motion; if they go to their end range, they may bypass the whole thing. But if they stay at 80 percent, they start to feel the tension across their muscles. All of a sudden, they're like, "Oh! That's what a muscle stretch feels like!" As hypermobile people, we often have to completely relearn how to be in our bodies.

These techniques all encourage interoceptive awareness as well. Interoception is the ability to sense inner physiological states. In the chapter "Common Bendy Body Complaints," I discussed how bendy people had been shown to have heightened interoceptive sensitivity (Eccles et al. 2012). This means their sense of changing physiological states can be distorted, inaccurate, and often overwhelming.

Gaining interoceptive clarity is critical to our ability to know how we feel, not only from a physiological perspective but also from an emotional perspective. The shifting emotional landscape we all experience moment to moment is also a sensory experience. Emotions bring changes to our inner physiological state. Some emotions bring a clenching to the belly, heat in the neck and face, a pounding or racing heart, or a tingle of joy.

As we learn to identify sensations and understand them as information coming to us from inside the body, we can better understand our emotional experiences as well. This is profoundly impactful for our ability to understand how we feel about various life situations, be able to communicate clearly, and hence, build stronger and more fulfilling connections with others.

AWARENESS OF OUR PARTS

Just as we can use verbal cues to guide students' awareness inward in the ways mentioned above, it can also be very useful to guide attention to specific parts of the body during asana practice. In the chapter "Common Bendy Body Complaints," I mentioned that people with hypermobility don't always have the best proprioception, and their brain's sensory "body map" may be a bit blurry. Developing specific awareness of the body during asana practice is one way to help the brain refine its map of the body and get more clarity on what's what.

Let's imagine I'm a bendy yoga student in a class, and I'm in Warrior II posture. I'm performing the posture just fine, but in my mind, I'm making my grocery list or rehashing a conversation I had earlier. But then the teacher cues me to notice my left big toe. Suddenly my brain makes contact with my left big toe, and I'm curious about how it feels. Then the teacher tells me to notice my right fingers, and suddenly my brain makes contact there. Next, the teacher might ask me to bring awareness to my left big toe and my right fingers simultaneously.

Before you know it, my awareness has landed smack dab in my body in the present moment. Now, I'm starting to notice what it feels like to be me. Well done, yoga teacher!

Teachers can also help students improve their awareness of specific body parts by describing the areas of the body that are contracting or stretching in a particular posture. In the chapter "Strength and Stability," I discussed how bendy people are master compensators. They can get a task done, but their brains may not recruit the right muscles to get it done optimally or efficiently. Directing their attention to specific body parts can be helpful in this regard.

However, as I also discussed in "Strength and Stability," even if a teacher accurately identifies the target muscle for the task at hand, some bendy people will still have trouble connecting to it in their bodies. Many will need external feedback to help them make contact with the target muscle or muscle group.

In our recent conversation, Trina Altman described how hard verbal cues were for her to make sense of when she started taking yoga classes.

For me, as a person who's hypermobile coming to yoga, none of the cues made sense because they were all internal. They were all like, "Engage this muscle or that muscle." And I was like, "I don't know how to use my brain to tell that muscle to engage." I needed resistance.

When a verbal cue doesn't quite cut it, students may need some external feedback from props, a wall, or even a "target practice" hands-on assist, which I'll discuss in the next chapter, "Hands-On Assists."

Trina now uses a lot of tricks to give her students the resistance many of them need to feel muscles contracting. Once they learn how it feels to contract the target muscle, they have an easier time connecting to it in a yoga posture. She shared a strategy she uses to help students learn to retract their shoulder blades or pull them toward each other.

In my class, I will have students pair up with a partner and do a little tug of war with a blanket. I'll say, "When you're pulling, that's your shoulder blades retracting. Can you feel the muscles required to do that?" Because a lot of times, activating muscles on the backside of your body without actually pulling a load is tough, especially for hypermobile people.

I must emphasize again: if you're a yoga teacher and you want to be able to direct your students' attention in these ways, you need a strong foundation in basic muscular anatomy. If you don't understand how the body works, it's hard to guide your students accordingly. This is one reason I am passionate about teaching anatomy to yoga instructors and helping them gain confidence speaking about the body through a monthly membership program called Anatomy Bites (www. AnatomyBites.com).

If you're a yoga teacher, unpacking your habitual verbal cues and language can transform your teaching. As you dig into the *why* of what you say, I hope you'll find clarity about what you want to communicate to your students. Language and verbal cues that invite people inward to investigate their experience, refine their body map, and even understand their compensatory habits are particularly helpful for bendy yoga practitioners. When we shift our language, asana becomes a tool for learning about and transforming our embodied experience.

If you're a practitioner, I hope this chapter has given you some new ways to "hear" the cues you are given in yoga classes that you attend. Perhaps you can create your own inner guidance about how you practice. When there's a cue to reach farther or go deeper, you can think to yourself, "Except for me. I'm going to stay right where I am." Trust that you don't need to stretch farther to be better and that all expressions of a posture are "full expressions." Your body is resilient, adaptable, and yours to explore.

CHAPTER 13:

Hands-On Assists

"I can't tell you how many stories I've heard of bendy yoga practitioners being injured while receiving a hands-on assist in yoga class."

Many yoga teachers use hands-on assists (also called adjustments) as a teaching tool in yoga class. This means they place their hands on students' bodies in an attempt to achieve a desired outcome. While a discussion about hands-on assists is relevant to any student population, it's particularly important for people with hypermobility.

Teachers should always get consent before placing their hands on students' bodies. There are many methods for letting students opt-in or opt-out of receiving hands-on assists. I attended a class once where the teacher handed out little cards to each student at the beginning of class. Each card was green on one side and red on the other. Students set out their cards with the green side up if they wanted assists and with the red side up if they didn't. As someone who doesn't prefer receiving hands-on assists, this method worked well for me.

Teachers use hands-on assists for a number of reasons. Some assists are used to "correct" a yoga posture, implying that achieving a certain version of a posture is the goal of practice. Other assists are used to push the student deeper into a posture, implying that going farther is better. These types of hands-on assists draw our attention externally toward a certain shape of the body.

Other times, assists are used to help students tune into an internal sensation. For example, some bring heightened awareness to a certain part of the body, while others offer a gentle massage to help a student relax while in a posture. Some assists suggest a direction of movement or elicit movement from within the student.

If you're a teacher, it's important to be clear about your intentions and approach students' bodies with reverence. If your assist is corrective in some way, you should have a good understanding of exactly why the pose needs fixing. If your assist aims to deepen a posture for a student, you should have a good understanding of why it's desirable to be in the posture more deeply.

I've received plenty of hands-on assists that made no sense to me and certainly didn't feel reverential. One such assist occurred while I was attending a yoga workshop in Missoula, Montana, in 2003. During one of our asana practices, the teacher lay down on top of me to deepen my seated forward fold.

A lot of things went through my mind in that moment. One of them was, "But, my face is already squished into my knees... where else can it go?" I didn't understand the point of the assist; it wasn't clear why going farther was desirable. The assist also felt violating. Placing hands on my lower back is one thing, but having the teacher lie down on top of me was certainly not what I had in mind.

Assists that deepen a student's posture are the most problematic for bendy people. I can't tell you how many stories I've heard of bendy yoga practitioners being injured while receiving a hands-on assist in yoga class.

Stepfanie Romine is a hypermobile yoga practitioner, teacher, and author living in Germany. She spent many years as an Ashtanga practitioner. Thanks to excellent instructors who helped her pay attention to her body and respect her unique needs as a bendy person, she evaded injury for a very long time. One day, she showed up to her usual Ashtanga class to learn a guest teacher would be teaching the class that day. She immediately felt apprehensive about doing the class with a teacher she didn't know. She decided to have a chat with the guest teacher before class and tell her about her hypermobility.

> I told her when I met her before class, "I have loose joints. My arms, especially, are very loose so please do not adjust them. Just don't try to adjust anything."

Stepfanie felt better about starting the practice after communicating her boundaries to the teacher. Unfortunately, during the course of the practice, the teacher adjusted her anyway. Worse still, she adjusted her arm, which Stepfanie had specifically warned her against. Perhaps she had forgotten about Stepfanie's request. Who knows? In any case, Stepfanie describes what happened.

> When we were in Marichyasana D, the teacher quickly grabbed my right forearm and yanked it around to get me deeper into the bind. It created an elbow ligament injury that took years to resolve. After that class, my elbow brace was a constant companion.

The posture Stepfanie was in when the teacher adjusted her arm position is difficult to envision if you're not familiar with it. You sit with one knee bent in front of you (cross-legged style) and the other knee bent up toward the sky. Then, you wrap your arms around to the sides, clasp your hands together behind your back, and twist (See Figure 13a).

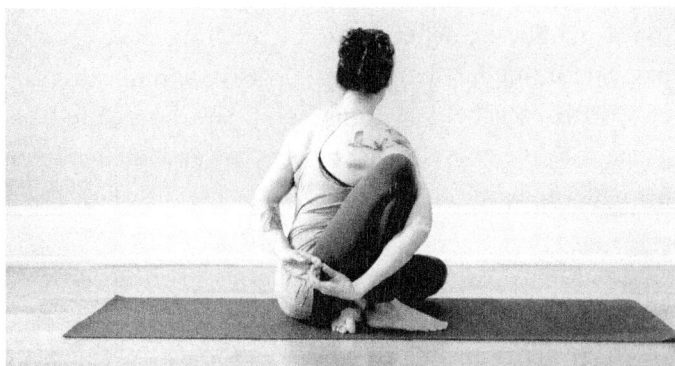

Figure 13a

The way the teacher adjusted Stepfanie in this posture caused long-lasting harm. It was also disempowering. Stepfanie set a clear boundary, and the teacher violated it. It's critical that as yoga teachers, we respect students' boundaries, not only to avoid injury but—just as importantly—to avoid disempowerment.

Melanie Downey, a bendy yoga and meditation teacher in Massachusetts, recently shared a story with me about a hands-on assist she received about eighteen years ago in a vinyasa yoga class.

> I remember it vividly. The teacher was young and over-zealous. She was blaring rock music throughout the class, so already I was overstimulated. She taught a lot of challenging postures, and I was certainly not one to shy away. At that point, I was still like, "I'm going to be the best one in this class!" Eventually we were in pigeon pose, and I had my front knee bent so my shin was at a comfortable angle. She walked over, grabbed my foot, and moved it so my front shin was parallel to the front of my mat. I heard a sound in my hip, and I was like, "Uh-Oh!" But I wanted to be cool, so I didn't say anything and I finished the class. I didn't realize the extent of my injuries until a couple days later, as often happens. And then I was flat out for like two weeks with hip and knee pain. I wish I never went to that class.

Melanie paints a familiar picture in describing this class: a fast-paced, challenging class in which students' attention is drawn outward by loud music, and the teacher's attention is focused on the shape of her students' bodies rather than their experience. As teachers, if we base our use of hands-on assists on an idea of how a posture is supposed to look, we completely override the experience of the practitioner. In that case, the assist may leave them feeling confused or, even worse, injured—as it did for Melanie that day.

Aside from being potentially injurious, assists that deepen a student's posture can interfere with the student's process of establishing their own movement boundaries. When I first learned how profound my own hypermobility was and understood how it was impacting my yoga-related injuries (this was long before my hEDS diagnosis), I started cultivating boundaries for my body by limiting my range of motion in asana practice.

Some bodies have a natural way of holding up an internal sign that says, "Stop here. You've gone far enough." My body didn't do this for me. Once I understood this was problematic, I learned to feel for any hint of sensation on my way into a pose. If I felt something, I practiced stopping right there. Even if I couldn't feel any sensation at all, I stopped short of my end range anyway.

One day, I was in a flow yoga class. We were in a standing forward fold with arms reaching behind our backs and hands clasped together (See Figure 13b). Given my history of chronic shoulder subluxation and injury, I had learned to reign this in. So, instead of stretching my arms as far as possible behind my back, I stopped at about half of my available range. While we were in that forward fold, the teacher came up and nonchalantly pushed my arms down toward the floor, pushing my shoulders about 30 degrees farther into extension.

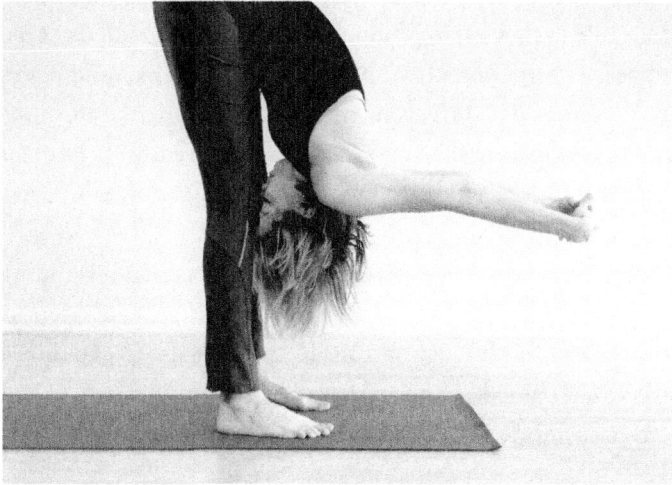

Figure 13b

I wasn't hurt, thank goodness, but I could have been. And aside from increasing my risk of injury, the teacher had unintentionally sent me a message about who's in charge of my body. There I was, working hard to create a boundary for myself, and the teacher just walked by and pushed my body past its boundary as if it was no big deal.

While there was no malice in this teacher's assist, there also wasn't a good reason for it. Again, if you're offering an assist to deepen someone's posture, making sure you have a good reason for thinking deeper is better.

Not all hands-on assists are problematic. The most helpful hands-on assists for bendy people are those that promote body awareness or elicit movement from within rather than imposing movement from outside.

These types of assists help students learn what the movement feels like so they can reproduce it on their own. I call this type of assist "target practice" because the teacher's hand essentially serves as a target for the student to breathe or move into. Having a target to push into is also incredibly helpful for proprioception. The resistance lets the body know where it is.

I received an assist like this once in a yoga class while standing in mountain pose. The teacher was bringing our awareness to the way the inhalation caused the rib cage to expand in the front, the sides, and the back. As a chronic sway-backed rib-thruster myself, this was a powerful inquiry for me.

The teacher came over and placed her hand on the back of my lower ribcage and said, "Breathe into my hand." Her hand made firm, clear contact with my body, and she used it to elicit something from within me. Her simple assist helped me feel the way my habitual posture impacted my breathing and how it felt to do it differently. The feeling of breathing into her hand was profound. I felt my lower ribs expand in the back, and the geometry of my entire body adjusted to a more comfortable and supported way to be upright.

Figures 13c and 13d show one way I might apply a "target practice" assist for downward dog at the wall if my intent was to encourage students to keep their spine long in a neutral position rather than dropping into a back bend. Figure 13c shows a hypermobile student flopping into a backbend and hyper flexing her shoulders, and 13d shows me using my hands to give her a target to push up into to achieve the desired position.

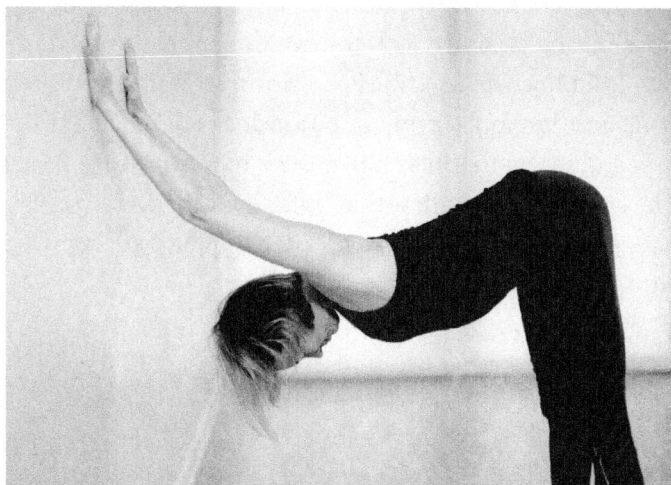

Figure 13c

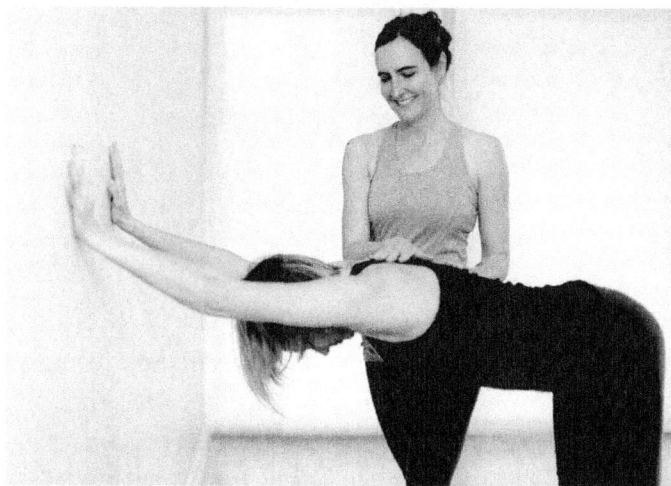

Figure 13d

For another example of how I use target practice assists, let's imagine a high lunge with the front knee bent. Sometimes the front knee drifts inward, collapsing toward the big toe. This isn't terribly alarming, but it does tell me about the wakefulness of the outer hip muscles in the front leg. When they're sleepy, they allow this "knee drift" to occur (See Figure 13e). Since I'm always interested in helping people develop strong hip muscles, this catches my eye.

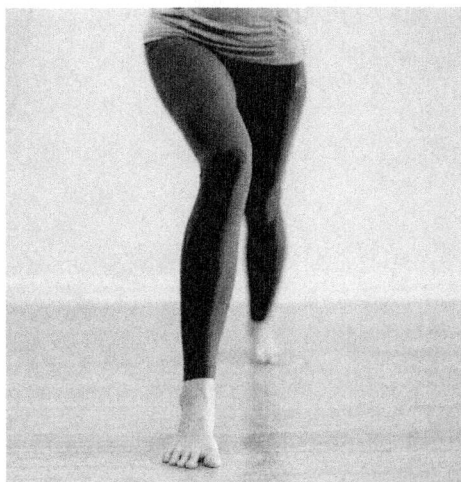

Figure 13e

When I see the knee drift, I will often walk over to my student, place my hand on the outer side of the front knee, and say, "Push your knee into my hand." What happens is hip abduction, which is accomplished by contracting the lateral hip muscles. The result is the front knee moves in the direction of the little toes (See Figure 13f).

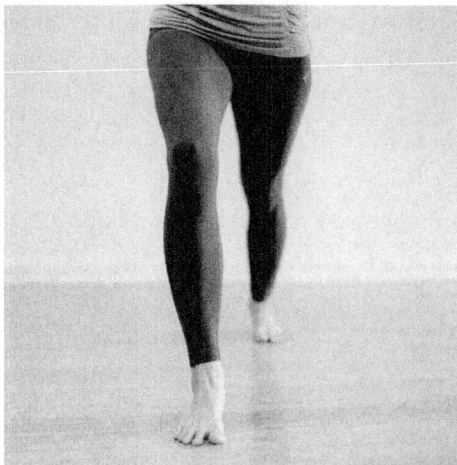

Figure 13f

I'm not concerned about the details of how far the knee actually moves. I'm interested in the student feeling the sensation of contracting her hip muscles. If I moved the student's knee there myself, the end result would look the same, but her inner experience wouldn't be the same at all. She wouldn't get the feeling of how to do it herself.

Keep in mind: if my verbal cues are effective, my students won't likely need a hands-on assist. For example, when the knee drift catches my eye in a high lunge, I might say something like, "See what it feels like to press your front knee out in the direction of your little toes." If the student still has trouble feeling what I'm talking about, a target practice assist can bring awareness to that part of the body and help the practitioner learn to do something new for herself. I find these assists incredibly empowering.

When it comes to hands-on assists, I believe "less is more." A little bit goes a long way. When used wisely, hands-on assists can serve to promote awareness, empowerment, and ease for the practitioner.

Just like language and verbal cues, hands-on assists are powerful. If you're a teacher, I hope this chapter gave you some helpful considerations for your use of hands-on assists. I encourage you to see and approach your students' bodies with reverence so that your assists (if any) leave students feeling safe and empowered. If you're a student, I hope you've gained insight into the types of assists you would consent to receive. And I encourage you to accept nothing less than reverence from your teacher.

PART 3:

BEYOND ASANA

CHAPTER 14:

Self-Massage

"This is not a wrestling match. This is a conversation with your nervous system."

One day years ago, I was teaching a group of yoga teachers-to-be. The students had just returned from their lunch break, and we had a few minutes before our session began. Students were milling about, practicing postures, chatting, and starting to gather for the afternoon session.

A young female student was doing a bit of stretching on the floor. Before I knew it, she had flopped herself easily into a deep split. Once in her split, she said to the classmate sitting next to her, "Ugh, my hamstrings are so tight!" The image of a bendy yoga practitioner complaining of tight hamstrings while in a deep split captures a bizarre phenomenon.

Bendy people feel "tight."

Muscle tension and pain is something I treat in nearly 100 percent of my hypermobile patients. It is often *the thing* driving their physical pain. In the chapter "Common Bendy Body Complaints," I discussed a few reasons bendy people feel tight. Those included chronic muscle contraction to compensate for lack of connective tissue support, postural habits, and increased sympathetic nervous system arousal.

In this chapter, I want to explore self-massage as a tool for finding relief. Self-massage techniques can be a fabulous adjunct to yoga practice, and if you're a teacher, they can add a whole new dimension to your class.

SELF-MASSAGE

Self-massage (or self-myofascial release, as it's sometimes called) is *the* practice that's had the most impact on my chronic myofascial pain. It simply means applying massage to your own body using some sort of tool. Many people use self-massage to relieve pain and tension, encourage layers of fascia to stay hydrated and mobile, or simply to relax. Tools include foam rollers, theracanes, therapy balls, and others. My favorite tools are therapy balls.

A variety of self-massage therapy balls are available on the market, but they don't have to be fancy to be effective. I've used tennis balls, racket balls, and even hand balls with good results. Some people prefer softer inflatable therapy balls; some prefer smaller, larger, or harder types of therapy balls. I encourage you to try a few different types to find the specific tools your body likes best.

Depending on your familiarity with muscular anatomy, it can be helpful to get some guidance or training on using therapy balls. While I'm introducing you to some basic concepts, I highly recommend Jill Miller's book *The Roll Model* for exploring it on your own (Miller 2014).

One of my favorite techniques is to place two tennis balls (or other similarly sized therapy balls) under my back such that they straddle my spine, with each ball making contact with the squishy muscle tissue on either side (See Figure 14a). Then, I roll them up and down my spine to massage my back muscles (See Figure 14b).

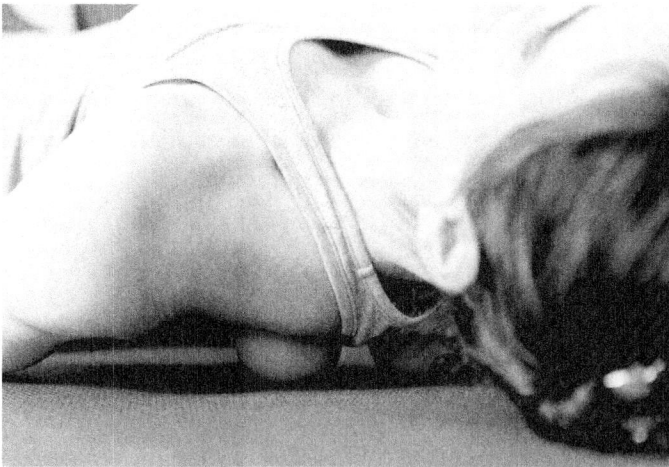

Figure 14a

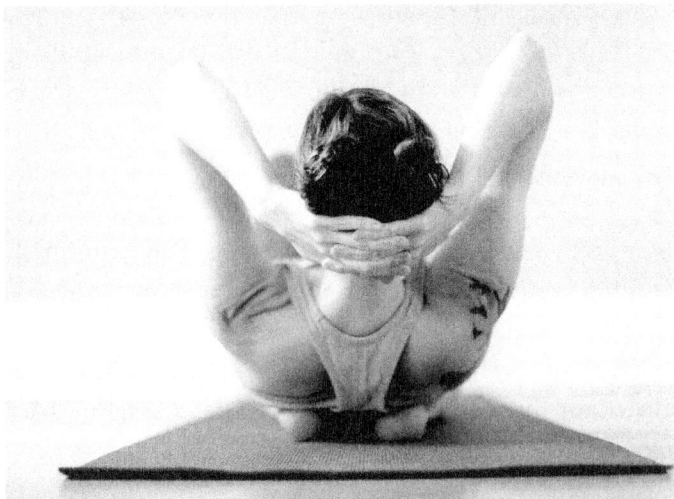

Figure 14b

I usually do this technique on the floor, but it can also be done leaning against a wall to decrease the pressure and sensation intensity. We all prefer different intensities of sensation, and finding the amount of pressure that feels good is key. Once you find the right amount of pressure, you lean in, relax, and enjoy for several minutes.

Be aware, some contraindications do apply for self-massage, including massaging over wounds and fractures. Caution is also warranted in the case of tissue inflammation, blood clots, and other conditions, including osteomyelitis and myositis ossificans (Bartsch et al. 2021). When in doubt, ask your doctor if massage presents any risks in your specific situation.

WHAT'S GREAT ABOUT IT

I use self-massage in my own self-care routine for many reasons. First of all, it allows me to scratch my muscle tension itch without stretching to my end ranges. Secondly, it invariably leaves me feeling more relaxed and centered afterward. Finally, thanks to its cost-effectiveness, I can reap the benefits of massage as frequently as I'd like after a one-time purchase of therapy balls (or any other tool of choice).

Research supporting self-massage for a variety of outcomes is growing, and more will likely emerge in the coming years. It has been shown to be effective at improving flexibility and muscle performance (Capobianco et al. 2019). It can also improve blood flow to tissues, helping to flush out cellular waste products that accumulate in chronically contracted muscle tissue (Soares et al. 2020). Research also suggests self-massage can reduce muscle pain (Wiewelhove et al. 2019), including in people with fibromyalgia (Ceca et al. 2017), and can even improve sleep quality (Kovaleva and Kovalev 2019).

General massage has been shown to facilitate relaxation and calming of the nervous system. Pressure stimulates mechanoreceptors within myofascial tissue, leading to decreased sympathetic nervous system arousal. In other words, massage can shift the autonomic nervous system into a calmer state (Barreto and Batista 2017; Morikawa et al. 2017; Shleip 2003). Many report the same experience of calm following self-massage.

Self-massage can also leave you with improved proprioception, whether you use it before or after exercise (David et al. 2019; Shin and Sung 2015). This is particularly relevant for bendy people who tend to struggle with accurately sensing their body's position in space (Clayton et al. 2015). Incorporating self-massage at the beginning of your asana practice can be a useful tool to help you "arrive" in your body for practice. In our recent conversation, Jill Miller emphasized this benefit of self-massage:

> A really beautiful thing about the balls is that they are always there to give you some feedback within the neural network from skin to bone, and that's going to give you an immediate knowing of where you are in space. When you take the ball away, you still feel that touch. And that ghost touch for the hypermobile person is so valuable for locating tissues. It's that self-locating that's going to keep you safe in asana practice.

Self-massage has also been shown to decrease delayed onset muscle soreness (Cheatham et al. 2015) and post-exercise fatigue (Schroeder and Best 2015). Because delayed onset muscle soreness can significantly limit bendy people's exercise tolerance, this is a wonderful reason to incorporate self-massage following your asana practice.

As always, the best research on self-massage is the research you do on yourself as you explore your own body and its response to the practice.

YOUR APPROACH IS EVERYTHING

The most important thing I tell my students and patients about self-massage is, "This is not a wrestling match. It's a conversation with your nervous system." It can be easy to approach the body aggressively as if we could hammer the tension away with forceful grimacing and grunting. This approach is like having a wrestling match with your body, and it doesn't usually go well.

Since resting muscle tone is largely influenced by your nervous system, an aggressive approach to the body can trigger a reactive increase in tension rather than a release. Remember, when the nervous system senses a threat, it creates muscle tension, which will be counterproductive to your goals.

Instead, I recommend approaching self-massage as though it's a conversation with your nervous system. Go into the body with a sense of curiosity like you're embarking on an adventure. Tune into the various qualities of sensation you find and notice how they change over time. Most importantly, be curious about your response to sensation. Do you tend to brace against it, or do you melt right into it? Some people like a lot of pressure and sensation; others don't.

Feeling safe is the key to a positive self-massage experience. Your breath will often be your first clue about how your nervous system is responding. When you feel safe, you'll notice that it's easier to maintain a long steady breath, following the exhale all the way to the end. You'll also be able to relax into the sensation. You'll notice your heart rate doesn't increase, your jaw doesn't tighten, and your face doesn't grimace.

Sometimes it takes a couple of minutes to adjust to the pressure of the self-massage tool and soften your body around it. I encourage people to stay with it for a few minutes to explore how the nervous system responds and adjusts.

When you don't feel safe, your breath may be choppy and shallow. Your heart may be racing. You may feel your body brace against the pressure, unable to relax. Perhaps your face is grimacing or your jaw clenching. These are all signs to instead change techniques, decrease the pressure, use a softer ball, or stop altogether. There are always techniques available to turn the sensation intensity up or down, so you stay within a zone that feels safe.

For example, if you're practicing a technique on the floor with your body weight on the therapy balls and the sensation is too great to relax into, try leaning against a wall instead so you can turn down the intensity. One of the most powerful aspects of self-massage is that it puts control in the hands of the user, empowering each individual to study their experience and make changes where necessary.

Words of guidance I consistently repeat to my students and patients include: "You're in charge of your body. You're in charge of the pressure and the sensation. And you're in charge of making changes where necessary to get comfortable. I'm here to help. Keep coming back to your breath as your guide. You don't get extra points for suffering."

I used to teach a weekly class dedicated to self-massage. I'd bring a big bag of therapy balls and lead the class through about forty-five minutes of self-massage on a specific area of the body. Then, we would finish with a few stretches and a long relaxation. Some students were visibly blissed out during class; others weren't quite sure about it.

I did my best to educate students about self-massage and help them understand that we all have different responses to pressure and sensation. I emphasized that part of what we are doing here is learning about those responses so we can better understand ourselves and find tools that feel good.

One day, a student who was new to self-massage came to class. As we got into the practice, I noticed she was grunting and grimacing. When I offered alternative techniques to turn down the sensation, she did not seem interested. She was clearly in a wrestling match with her body.

I went over to the student and said, "How's it going over here?" She replied with a grimace, "Is this supposed to hurt?" I replied, "Well, I certainly expect you to have some interesting sensations! Tell me more about what you are feeling." We proceeded to have a conversation about what she was feeling. Turning her attention toward the sensations to examine and describe them in more detail seemed to calm her down.

I told her that even though it's safe to press on her tissues (barring contraindications), it often brings up intense sensations. I reminded her she was in charge of all the sensations in her body and that I'd be glad to help her find techniques that feel better. She finally agreed to try some techniques to turn down the intensity, which allowed her to relax into the experience.

I saw her whole approach change. She was finally having a conversation with her system, rather than a wrestling match. Taking charge of her experience and making changes to get more comfortable helped her feel empowered and safe.

When we have discomfort in the body, an understandable response is to turn away from, avoid, and brace ourselves against the sensations. Unfortunately, that can create more muscle tension and, in turn, more pain. If we can find ways *that feel safe* to turn toward and be with sensation rather than resisting it, we have an opportunity to change our relationship with it.

Self-massage is one such tool. This is not to say everyone will eventually like it. Some people don't, and it's not a character flaw. I encourage you to explore self-massage to find out if it's a useful tool for your body. If you're a teacher, consider incorporating a couple of techniques into your asana classes and see how your students respond. Self-massage can truly be a practice of self-study to develop awareness about your unique body, investigate your habitual response to sensation, and study your beliefs about discomfort, your body's potential, and yourself.

CHAPTER 15:

Calming the Nervous System

"Pranayama practice can help us deepen our relationship with, and better regulate, our nervous system to optimize physiological resilience."

In the previous chapters, I focused on the third limb of yoga (asana) and explored techniques most relevant for the bendy yoga practitioner. Asana is most directly related to musculoskeletal integrity and well-being, with features such as motor control, mindful stretching, stability, and postural awareness being particularly important for bendy people. Certainly, much of the bendy person's physical discomfort can be addressed through movement-based approaches, including asana practice.

As we explore our physical experience through asana, we also become more aware of inner sensations, also referred to as interoceptive signals, which tell us about our physiology and give us a direct line to the state of the nervous system.

A great deal of the bendy person's discomfort is related to the hypervigilant nervous system, so common among people with hypermobility syndromes. In the chapter "Common Bendy Body Complaints," I discussed several factors that contribute to this phenomenon, including an enlarged amygdala, dysautonomia (difficulty regulating heart rate and blood pressure), and joint instability.

These factors, among others, can cause the nervous system of bendy people to chronically live in a heightened state of sympathetic arousal, leading to muscle tension, chronic pain, anxiety, and digestive problems—some of the most common bendy body complaints. To better understand what this means, let's review some nervous system basics.

NERVOUS SYSTEM BASICS

The nervous system consists of a central part (brain and spinal cord) and a peripheral part (spinal and peripheral nerves). It carries information back and forth between your body and your brain and regulates all aspects of functioning.

The peripheral nervous system consists of somatic and autonomic components. The somatic system is responsible for controlling voluntary activities such as movement. The autonomic nervous system controls automatic activities such as breathing, heart rate, and digestion.

Traditionally, the peripheral autonomic nervous system has been described as having two components—sympathetic and parasympathetic. The sympathetic portion is activated when we are threatened or perceive threats to our physical or emotional safety. It's responsible for mobilizing our energy and is often called the "fight or flight" mode. When activated, we have increased blood flow to the periphery of the body, dilation of the pupils, dilation of the bronchioles, higher heart rate, and increased blood pressure (Alshak and Das 2021).

The parasympathetic branch has been described as the "rest and digest" mode because it is active when we feel calm, safe, and connected to ourselves or others. In this mode, we have a lower heart rate, lower blood pressure, and increased activity of the digestive system (Alshak and Das 2021).

In recent years, our collective understanding of the autonomic nervous system has evolved, in large part thanks to the work of Dr. Stephen Porges, who developed the Polyvagal Theory in 1995 (Porges 1995). The Polyvagal Theory illuminates the role of the vagus nerve in regulating the autonomic nervous system and presents a more nuanced understanding of the various nervous system states we experience as we respond to life events moment to moment.

THE VAGUS NERVE

The vagus nerve is the primary component of the parasympathetic nervous system. It is the tenth cranial nerve and the longest nerve of the body, meandering from the brainstem all the way to the abdomen. Along the way, it innervates the heart and digestive tract, in addition to parts of the ears, throat, and vocal cords (Porges 1995).

When stimulated, the vagus nerve dampens sympathetic arousal. In other words, it turns down the "fight or flight" response by lowering heart rate and blood pressure (Porges 2009). Because of this, the vagus nerve's effect on heart rate is sometimes referred to as the "vagal brake" (Dana 2018).

To complicate matters, the vagus nerve has two different components—a dorsal (toward the back) part that emerges from one place in the brain and a ventral (toward the front) part that emerges from a different place. Which part of the vagus nerve is activated—dorsal or ventral—will determine the quality of autonomic response (Dana 2018).

While we used to consider two autonomic nervous system states (sympathetic and parasympathetic), Polyvagal Theory suggests we actually have three: sympathetic, dorsal vagal, and ventral vagal (Dana 2018).

Sympathetic arousal is just as I described earlier—it is the "fight or flight" mode that helps us take action in the face of threat. Think of this as mobilized energy, like what you feel when you're so fired up you want to go to battle about something.

The dorsal vagal response emerges when the dorsal (toward the back) part of the vagus nerve is stimulated. We could describe this as a "collapsed" state. It's the nervous system's response to life-threatening danger when no escape seems possible. It is characterized by immobilization, such as you might feel when a situation is so overwhelming you just want to curl up into a ball and disappear.

Lastly, the ventral vagal state occurs when the ventral (toward the front) part of the vagus nerve is stimulated. This is a state in which you feel safe, connected, and relaxed (Dana 2018). Think of this as balanced energy, like what you feel when you're in a cozy and comfortable place, engaged in a stimulating conversation with a dear friend. That's why the ventral vagus nerve is considered a key part of our "social engagement system." When we are in that state, we are able to engage meaningfully and authentically with those around us.

Sympathetic and dorsal vagal responses aren't always negative. They can also occur in conjunction with the ventral vagal state—something referred to as "hybrid" states (Rosenberg 2017). For example, sometimes, we are inspired by a new creative project or motivated to plan an exciting vacation. That's when we are experiencing safe mobilization. It's sympathetic activation that is anchored to the ventral vagal state.

Likewise, when we are resting deeply or experiencing intimacy with someone we trust, we are safely immobilized. It's dorsal vagal activation that is anchored to a ventral vagal state. The ability to stay anchored to the ventral vagal (balanced) state, or return to it once the threat of danger has passed, is commonly referred to as nervous system regulation.

The cues we pick up from those around us are important for nervous system regulation. Because the ventral vagus nerve is involved with our ears, facial expressions, and vocal cords, its activation is dependent on cues of safety or danger in the environment around us. That means the faces and voices of those around us are powerful cues that encourage or discourage our return to a ventral vagal state (Porges 2017).

If you're a yoga teacher, this brings up the importance of your tone of voice and facial expressions as a factor in helping your students feel safe and calm for practice, not to mention your choice of music (if any).

People with HSD/hEDS have been shown to have low vagal tone and efficiency, which essentially means the vagus nerve isn't functioning optimally (Kolacz et al. 2021). It isn't as good at putting the brakes on sympathetic arousal. This likely contributes to a wide variety of challenges, including the overactive sympathetic response associated with anxiety, alongside POTS (Postural Orthostatic Tachycardia Syndrome) and digestive issues (Kolacz et al. 2021). Low vagal tone is also associated with conditions such as Rheumatoid Arthritis, Irritable Bowel Syndrome, and Inflammatory Bowel Disease (Bonaz et al. 2016).

Stimulating the vagus nerve can improve vagal tone and efficiency. In turn, this can lead to improved health outcomes due in part to the vagus nerve's role in decreasing systemic inflammation (Bonaz et al. 2016). Improved vagus nerve function also leads to greater nervous system regulation (Laborde et al. 2017; Kovacic et al. 2020). Being better regulated makes it easier to stay anchored to the ventral vagus "social engagement system," where we can connect with others and form meaningful relationships.

So, how can bendy people (and others) improve the function of their vagus nerve for better nervous system regulation and health? There are many ways to improve vagal tone, and many are available to use in yoga practice. Movement, breathing, and sound are all simple ways. Below, we will explore breathing practices that can help us cultivate calm.

PRANAYAMA

The fourth limb of yoga, pranayama, refers to breath practices designed to nourish and balance the animating vital energy known as prana. In less yogic terms, we can think of pranayama practices as a direct way to nourish, balance, and otherwise influence the nervous system—which controls physiological function.

Pranayama practices influence or manipulate the breath for a desired effect. If you're a yoga teacher, you're likely familiar with a number of specific techniques. While we all respond to practices in our own ways, certain techniques are more likely to cultivate a calming response for the nervous system.

Breathing practices don't need to be fancy to be powerful. The simple act of deep, slow breathing, especially with a long exhale, stimulates the calming effect of the ventral vagus nerve. It is an ever-present tool to help us stay anchored in or return to a ventral vagal state (Bonaz et al. 2016).

In *The Pocket Guide to The Polyvagal Theory: The Transformative Power of Feeling Safe*, Stephen Porges states, "Pranayama yoga, functionally, is the yoga of the social engagement system..." precisely because the breath can be so effective at stimulating the ventral vagus nerve (Porges 2017). Two of my favorite pranayama practices for this purpose include ujjayi (victorious breath) and bhramari (bumblebee breath).

Ujjayi (victorious breath) involves constricting the vocal cords slightly as you breathe in and out of the nose. It feels a bit like whispering. The effect is an audible sound akin to an ocean wave. I often describe it as trying to fog up your bathroom mirror with your mouth closed.

Bhramari (bumblebee breath), in its simplest form, involves humming your exhale all the way to the end, thereby lengthening the exhale. The humming is an added benefit beyond the long exhale. Humming, chanting, singing, and even gargling can help to stimulate the vagus nerve.

The "releasing breath" is another simple technique that uses breath and sound to stimulate a calming response for the nervous system. It involves taking a long inhale through the nose, followed by an audible sigh out the mouth for the full duration of the exhale.

Fast-paced breathing practices, such as kapalabhati (skull shining breath) and bhastrika (bellows breath), are likely to produce a different effect. Skull shining breath involves a quick, forceful exhale followed by a quick passive inhale, whereas bellows breath involves quick, forceful inhales and exhales. Traditionally, both tend to stimulate increased sympathetic arousal, which may or may not be useful, depending on the practitioner's needs. For people who suffer from anxiety or panic disorder, such breathing practices can exacerbate those issues.

When exploring pranayama practices, rather than forcing the breath to be a certain way, I encourage practitioners to *invite* the breath to change in the intended way. If a long exhale is the goal, but we force the exhale to be as long as humanly possible, we may end up causing agitation rather than calm. Instead, if we invite, rather than force, the exhale to be as long as it can be comfortably, we will likely have better results.

We don't all respond the same way to the same pranayama practices. It can be helpful to start with some guiding principles, as I've described above. But it's always important to invite inquiry into the effect of each specific practice. Did it lead to increased feelings of calm? Did it lead to increased anxiety? Did it leave you feeling balanced? This is another example of how curiosity, rather than expectation, can help us learn about ourselves and lead to transformation.

One of my most challenging moments as a yoga teacher occurred when I was introducing a teacher training group to ujjayi pranayama (victorious breath), which I described above. I led the group through five to ten minutes of practice and then invited students to share their experiences. Some students shared that they felt energized by the practice; others felt sleepy. One felt calm and alert at the same time; another felt anxious.

I explained there is no right or wrong way to feel the effect of the practice, and the diverse experiences reported by the group showed how variable our response might be. One student raised her hand with a scowl on her face and said, "But what is it *supposed* to feel like?"

I responded, "There isn't a particular way it is supposed to feel. The practice may impact us all differently and might even impact the same person differently on different days. There isn't a specific right answer here."

This student was thoroughly unsatisfied with my response. She shot back, "But you're the teacher. You're supposed to know the answer. I came here for answers, and now it feels like I'm just wasting my money."

I was surprised by her anger toward me and a bit embarrassed by the outburst in front of the large group of students. I took a couple of deep breaths to calm my own nervous system and then explained that, like all the practices of yoga, the breathing technique is a tool to investigate your own experience. Even though we wish things were black and white, reality is usually more of a gray area.

Encouraging yourself (or your students) to pay close attention to the effects of a breathing practice can lead to a deeper relationship with the nervous system. When we learn which techniques leave us feeling calmer or more balanced inside, we can emphasize those techniques not only in our practice but also in everyday life, where nervous system regulation matters even more.

Traditionally, pranayama techniques are practiced in a seated position following asana practice. However, pranayama does not exclusively have to be performed separately from asana. In fact, asana practice is a great place to incorporate breathing techniques. For example, in a style of asana where you perform slow, dynamic movement matched to the pace of your breath, the whole practice becomes a moving pranayama practice. Allowing the pace of your movement to match a slow, steady breath also brings a rhythmic quality to practice which can be soothing in its own right.

Sometimes, I incorporate bhramari pranayama (bumblebee breath) or mantra chanting into asana practice. I enjoy matching the sound-filled exhale to my movements, especially in simple postures. For example, while lying on my back, I like to use the entire length of my inhale to take my arms overhead behind me and then use the length of the exhale to bring them back down to my sides (See Figure 15a). This is an easy place to incorporate the humming bhramari breath, or even a simple mantra, on the exhales.

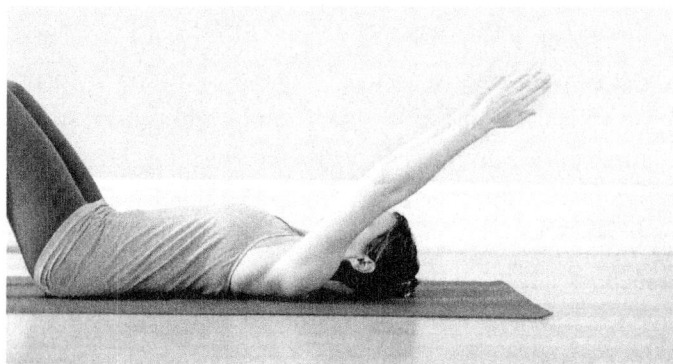

Figure 15a

Many yoga teachers pace their students' breathing during asana or pranayama practice. For example, they may say something like, "Inhale for 1, 2, 3, 4. Exhale for 1, 2, 3, 4," and so on. This is problematic because we all have naturally varying breath paces. It's hard for some students to stay in sync with the teacher's prescribed breath pace. Some end up breathing faster or slower than is comfortable. Either way, it can be agitating to the system. I like to encourage students to breathe (and move) at their own pace whenever possible.

Pranayama practice is a tool that prepares the practitioner for meditation. When our nervous system is dysregulated or agitated, it's more difficult to focus the mind for meditation, which I'll discuss in the next chapter, "Focusing the Mind."

Before we get there, I want to discuss a few other ways we can facilitate deep calm for the nervous system in yoga practice. These include relaxation, restorative postures, and weighted objects.

OTHER SIMPLE PRACTICES FOR CALM

The final pose of most asana practices is savasana or corpse pose. This is when you lie down comfortably and rest (See Figure 15b). It's an important time to reflect on the practice, let go of any lingering effort, and allow the benefits of the practice to settle in. Unfortunately, it's not uncommon to get a mere five minutes in savasana at the end of class. I encourage you to try spending ten to fifteen minutes in your final relaxation at the end of your asana practice and notice the difference it makes for you.

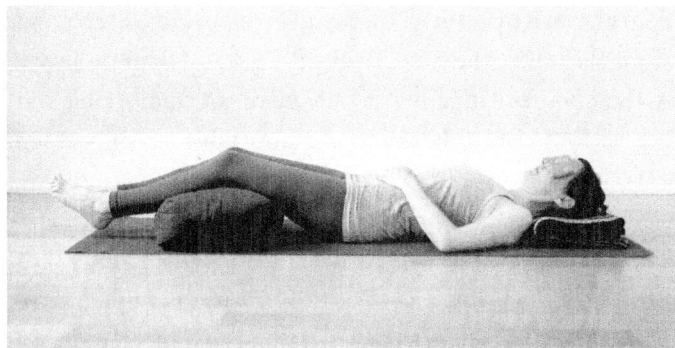

Figure 15b

Restorative yoga is another excellent resource for bringing a sense of calm to the nervous system. Rather than producing a strong sense of stretch, restorative postures place your body in various comfortable positions for relaxation. Your body is well supported by props such as bolsters, blankets, or blocks, and you stay for up to twenty minutes or longer (See Figure 15c). Much like corpse pose, there's nothing to do in these postures except rest. Some practitioners like to incorporate simple pranayama or visualization techniques while in restorative postures to help cultivate inner awareness and calm.

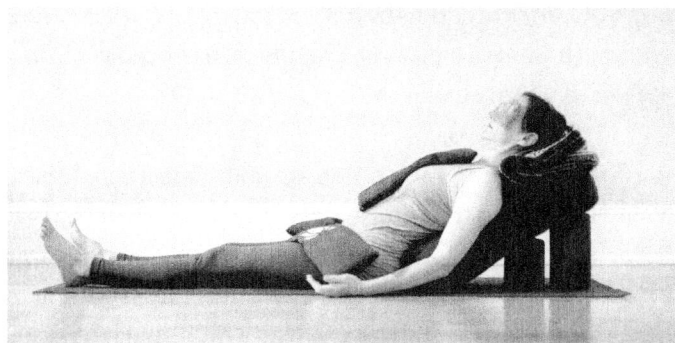

Figure 15c

For restorative postures, the setup is important. I encourage students to take the time necessary to set up their props well so their bodies can fully relax. If you're not comfortable starting out, you certainly won't be comfortable ten minutes in.

Corpse pose and restorative postures give people a chance to learn what it feels like to be awake and relaxed at the same time, to take a break, and to be fully present with themselves. It's not uncommon for people to fall asleep during these postures, and that's okay—it probably means they need more sleep! But relaxing in an awake state can have a powerful effect on the nervous system.

Weighted objects in the form of sandbags (a yoga prop commonly available in yoga studios), weighted blankets, eye pillows, or other similar products are also useful tools for bendy practitioners. A weighted object on their body provides a sense of deep but comfortable pressure that many enjoy during corpse pose or any restorative posture (See figure 15c).

Deep pressure can induce a calming effect for the nervous system (Reynolds et al. 2015). It is also commonly used to improve proprioceptive awareness and overall sensory integration (Bodison et al. 2018). I highly recommend exploring the use of weighted objects.

While the wonders of relaxation are many, most people have a hard time going from full speed to total relaxation in a matter of minutes. An active asana practice can help discharge extra energy and prepare us for relaxation. Especially for someone who's feeling anxious, doing a more dynamic asana practice first can improve the effectiveness of the relaxation.

Exploring pranayama practice and various methods of relaxation can be enormously helpful for bendy people. Nichi Linder, a yoga teacher with hEDS in Springfield, Oregon, talks about how important the calming aspects of yoga practice have been for her to manage her symptoms.

Yoga offers so much to calm down the sympathetic nervous system activation that folks with EDS, fibromyalgia, and anyone in chronic pain, deal with. To me, that is the place where yoga can be super helpful. My practice has become heavily focused on pranayama, relaxation, and meditation, in addition to gentle strengthening.

Each of the eight limbs of yoga is designed to move us along a continuum of practices from gross to subtle. We began with asana practice, which can help us cultivate a deeper relationship with our body and, in turn, lead to improved physical resilience.

In this chapter, we have explored how pranayama practice and relaxation techniques can help us deepen our relationship with and better regulate our nervous system to optimize physiological resilience. When we are able to regulate our nervous system states, many good things happen. We support overall physiological health, make ourselves available for meaningful connection with others, and calm down enough for the meditative practices I'll discuss in the next chapter.

CHAPTER 16:

Focusing the Mind

"Yoga can help you start to see yourself and the purpose of your life with more clarity and understand that you're not your disease."

— KRISTINE KAOVERII WEBER

Up to this point, we have explored how asana and pranayama can best support bendy people. Physical postures allow us to feel sensations and learn what the body needs. Breathing techniques can help relieve stress and be an anchor for awareness. In the context of Patanjali's eight limbs of yoga discussed in the chapter, "What is Yoga?" asana and pranayama prepare us for the meditative practices of the last four limbs.

The last four limbs of yoga include pratyahara (withdrawal of the senses), dharana (concentration), dhyana (meditation), and samadhi (absorption or union). These meditative practices can lead to a deeper understanding of ourselves, our connection to the world around us, and to something greater. Meditative practices can be supportive for bendy people for a number of reasons I'll discuss in this chapter.

The fifth limb of yoga, pratyahara, is the withdrawal of the senses. This means focusing attention inward, away from the external world of sensory stimulation. It represents the first step in meditation.

Quieting the body through asana and quieting the breath through pranayama can help facilitate pratyahara in which the practitioner becomes still, closes the eyes, and reduces sound and other sensory stimulation as much as possible. Pratyahara can give an overwhelmed sensory system the rest and reset it needs in addition to preparing us for concentration practices.

Once we gather our awareness inward, we can move into the sixth limb of yoga, dharana, which is concentration. Concentration focuses attention on one object, whether that object is a part of the body, the breath, an image, or a mantra. Concentration is essentially a "warm-up" for meditation.

The seventh limb of yoga is dhyana, which means meditation or contemplation. This is essentially the state of being resulting from sustained concentration. Through sustained attention on an object, the practitioner is said to come to a deeper understanding of the object and of themselves. Ultimately, the idea is that the practitioner becomes completely absorbed in the nature of the object on which they are meditating. Many people describe it as being "in the zone."

Whereas concentration requires effort, the state of dhyana or meditation feels effortless.

The eighth limb of yoga is samadhi, which is described as a state of absorption or union that may be achieved through meditation. It arises for brief moments (or longer) when the practitioner fully understands and merges with the object of meditation. It's like being completely connected to the higher self or some sense of the Divine.

What I've given you above is a brief description of the steps toward meditation that Patanjali described in the *Yoga Sutras*. Think of it as a road map. The idea is that through consistent practice, the practitioner may have glimpses of those states of being "in the zone" or being completely connected to something greater than themselves. But as is the case with all of yoga practice, the tools are just tools. Where they lead us will vary from person to person and day to day.

More broadly speaking, meditation is a term that is defined in a variety of ways. While meditation techniques vary, they share a common intention: training the practitioner's mind toward a higher goal. In the yoga tradition, a simple way of describing meditation is to call it "attention training." Most traditional yogic meditation techniques focus the attention on a singular object, mantra, or image.

Mindfulness meditation, which comes out of the Buddhist tradition, cultivates an expansive awareness of the comings and goings of thoughts and feelings. It's a practice of observing ourselves from a place of acceptance and curiosity.

Through practice, we improve our ability to witness our experiences with kindness.

There is no one "right" way to meditate. It's a good idea to try out various techniques to determine what you like. But when you find one you like, it's good to stick with it for a while because consistency, rather than the specific technique, is what generally leads to transformation.

Start with five minutes, and over time, you may find you are able to practice for longer. There's also no "right" position for meditation, even though it is traditionally done in a seated position. Bendy people may need alternative positioning, in particular due to Orthostatic Intolerance (difficulty being upright) associated with dysautonomia (difficulty regulating heart rate and blood pressure). These challenges lead many to experience dizziness, fast heart rate, shortness of breath, fatigue, agitation, or other forms of discomfort during prolonged sitting.

I've talked with some yoga practitioners who are committed to a seated upright position as the only right way to meditate. While I understand there is a quality of alertness that comes with being upright, for those with Orthostatic Intolerance, an alternative position might be more suited for their needs.

Nichi Linder, a yoga teacher with hEDS, has found meditation helpful in her practice. However, she also shared her struggle to find a comfortable position due to Orthostatic Intolerance and low back pain. Like Nichi, many bendy people find upright seated meditation uncomfortable, if not intolerable. She explained:

I decided at some point I could lie down for meditation and the gods of meditation were not going to frown upon me. If it's the difference between not meditating at all, or meditating lying down, I'd rather lie down.

The discomfort of being upright can be a significant distraction to the practice of meditation. Melanie Downey, a bendy yoga and meditation teacher, shared a similar experience.

I first started meditating in college in the early nineties with a Buddhist group that came to campus when I was eighteen or nineteen years old. I knew I had hypermobile joints but didn't really understand what that meant. I'd already had multiple knee surgeries. My back and neck, my hips and feet—everything was always sore. For meditation, we would sit and focus on the breath, and every minute a bell would sound to refocus our breathing. I loved it, so I stuck with it. Everyone else seemed to be able to sit and do their thing, but I would develop all this pain and I'd always have to be fidgeting. It wasn't until five or six years later that I was told it was okay to lie down. Then, everything changed for me. We have this idea in our mind that it's got to be a certain way, but really, there are thousands of ways to meditate. All we're looking to do is still the mind. Any way you can accomplish that gets the job done.

Lying down or being supported in a reclining or semi-reclining position may allow more access to inner experience (See Figure 16a). I encourage you to find a position that is comfortable for you so you can enjoy some of the potential benefits of meditation.

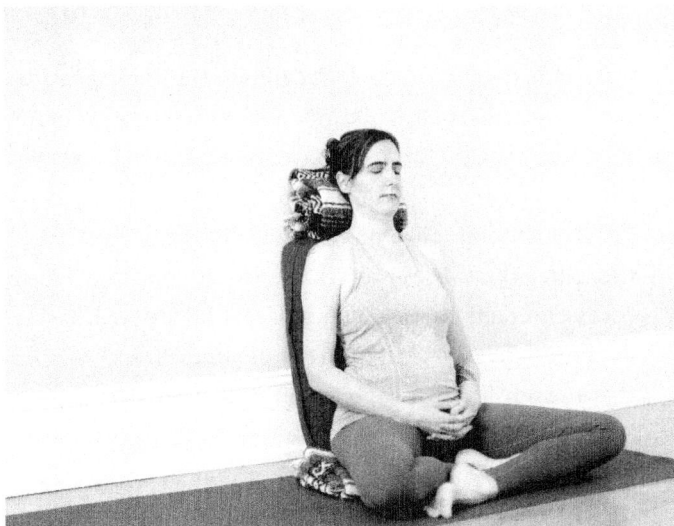

Figure 16a

I've had many students complain to me that "they can't meditate" because their mind keeps wandering from thought to thought and never seems to calm down. I tell them meditation is simply a way to practice paying attention. Through practice, our ability to pay attention gets stronger. But the mind will indeed wander, some days more than others. When you notice your mind wandering, it's okay. Simply invite your focus back to the object of meditation with kindness and self-compassion. Then, repeat over and over again. It can feel like push and pull sometimes, but that's the practice.

I've also talked to a lot of yoga teachers who feel stressed over not meditating enough. They think if they could just check that hour of meditation per day off their list, they will have arrived at being a good yoga teacher. Meditation isn't a performance, and it's not something to mark off your to-do list. Rather, it's time away from your to-do list. More consistent practice will amplify the benefits, but whether it's five minutes per week or thirty minutes per day, meditation is a way home to yourself.

Stepping back to witness ourselves in this way can lead to greater self-awareness and self-compassion. Such practices can help practitioners understand and reframe habits of thought and behavior that may or may not be serving their life goals. Sometimes, meditation can reveal aspects of our relationship with ourselves that would be hard to see otherwise.

This was the case for me when I started meditating. Even though I was physically active in sports during childhood, I managed to escape the discomfort of my body to some degree. Without meditation, I may not have ever discovered that I'd been having a bit of an "out of body experience."

In my early twenties, I went to graduate school at the University of Montana to study Environmental Studies. This was long before I became a yoga instructor and then a physical therapist. While I enjoyed a lot of things about my time in Montana, it was also the time when my anxiety and depression became more severe, and I decided to start therapy. I was lucky to find a therapist who introduced me to mindfulness meditation, and it changed my life.

She put me through the Mindfulness-Based Stress Reduction program developed by Jon Kabat-Zinn. There was nothing easy about it. Nonetheless, I did my homework and developed a daily meditation practice. It revealed something surprising about my relationship with my body.

For nearly a year, each time I sat for meditation, I never felt like I was actually inhabiting my body. Instead, I seemed to observe myself from somewhere above. I couldn't figure out how to get down there and be in my body.

Over time, these practices did help me find my way back to my body during meditation. Eventually, my perspective shifted. Instead of watching myself meditate, I was doing the meditating. I still remember the giddy, triumphant feeling I had when I first noticed the change.

Reflecting on that experience, I think my return to my body required me to first understand that inner sensations are safe to notice and experience. When we don't understand what's happening in our bodies, it's easy to turn away from the discomfort in fear.

Changing my relationship with discomfort helped me turn toward my experience, develop curiosity about it, and finally learn about it. In my case, meditation helped me learn about *me*—my body, my thoughts, my feelings, and my habits. Meditation became an avenue to connect with my higher self that has perspective and can witness my circumstances with compassion. It gave me a feeling of a supportive presence in my life. From there, it has become easier to learn how to take care of myself.

The benefits of meditation are well documented, and bendy people are more likely to struggle with several challenges that meditation has been shown to ameliorate. People with hypermobility show characteristic atypical brain structures, including an enlarged amygdala, contributing to anxiety, and a smaller parietal cortex, contributing to deficits in proprioception (sense of joint position and body awareness).

Various forms of meditation have been shown to induce changes that essentially reverse bendy people's atypical brain structure differences. For example, regular meditation has been shown to decrease the size of the amygdala (fear center in the brain) and increase the size of the parietal cortex, home of the brain's sensory body map (Froeliger et al. 2012).

Hypermobility is strongly correlated with ADHD (Glans et al. 2021). Preliminary research suggests mindfulness meditation can serve a supportive role for adults with ADHD, leading to reduction of some symptoms and improvement in emotional regulation (Mitchell et al. 2017).

Bendy people have also been shown to have altered interoception, which is the ability to sense internal physiological states. Specifically, the volume of those inner sensations is turned up so that they can become distorted and overwhelming, leading to an inaccurate interpretation of the signals coming from inside their bodies. To put it most simply, bendy people have a hard time knowing how they feel.

In our recent conversation, Kristine Kaoverii Weber, a yoga teacher and founder of Subtle Yoga, described the far-reaching ramifications of impaired interoception and how it leads right to the heart of yoga.

> Not knowing how we feel lies at the heart of so much of our suffering because those inner sensations often drive our behavior. We engage in so many behaviors because we ignore or don't understand the body's messages. Maybe I eat more because I don't feel good, and I don't know that I don't feel good. Maybe I'm not even aware I'm trying to fill this hole which might be emotional or physical pain, or it might be loneliness. But then I have to deal with the fallout of those behaviors for myself and others. When you're ignoring the messages your body's sending you, you're ignoring yourself and the deeper meaning and purpose of your life.

Some interesting research suggests meditation can lead to improved interoceptive accuracy (Daubenmier et al. 2013). This lends support to the idea that meditative practices can help bendy people learn to interpret their inner sensations more accurately and thereby develop a deeper relationship with themselves.

Once we learn about and understand how we feel, we have an opportunity to get support where necessary. From a place of clarity about who we are, we can take action, address our needs, and make better decisions about how we behave toward other people and ourselves.

In fact, regular yoga practice in general has been shown to improve several aspects of mental and cognitive function, including executive function. Executive function includes planning, decision-making, and cognitive flexibility, among other aspects (Gothe et al. 2018). Improvements can be appreciated even after a single yoga session (Gothe et al. 2013).

Melanie Downey describes how meditation helps her find her way to her True Self—a place of clarity that ultimately leads to more mindful behavior in life situations that are difficult.

For me, the end goal of meditation is to put us in a place where we're able to think clearly and objectively so we are able to control our reactions to everything around us. When something happens, you're able to say, "Okay, this happened." And without reacting from your senses, you can respond from a place of—I guess you could call it the True Self, stripped of external stimuli and our body's chemical responses to them— where you're able to behave in a way that is calm so you can make a proper decision.

FULL CIRCLE

Taking action based on a clearer understanding of ourselves brings us full circle to the first two limbs of yoga—the yamas (how to be nice to others) and niyamas (how to be nice to yourself). Yoga's ethical principles provide a framework that can guide optimal self-care for people with hypermobility syndromes. In addition to asana, pranayama, and meditation practices, consistent practice and reflection on the yamas and niyamas can also support optimal health.

The yamas include:

- ahimsa, or non-violence
- satya, or truthfulness
- asteya, or non-stealing
- brahmacarya, or moderation
- aparigraha, or non-hoarding

The niyamas include:

- sauca, or cleanliness
- samtosa, or contentment
- tapas, or inner effort
- svadhyaya, or self-study
- isvarapranidhana, or surrender to the Divine

When we consider the yamas and niyamas in the context of hypermobility syndromes, they can present us with reminders to practice asana in a way that reduces harm, be honest with ourselves and others about our unique needs, and set clear boundaries around our energy expenditure. They can guide us in taking optimal care of ourselves, becoming the experts on our own condition, and accepting ourselves and our unique life challenges just as they are.

Iryna Merideth is a bendy yoga practitioner and teacher living in Carrboro, North Carolina. During a recent conversation I had with her, she reflected on her experience of bendiness in the context of yoga. After working through some challenges related to her hypermobility, she eventually had to shift her approach to yoga from one of competition and performance to one of inner study and self-acceptance.

I've had to reflect a lot on what I'm after in yoga. Do I want to be *the best* in class by doing extreme postures that lead to pain the next day, or is this about something bigger? There's so much internal work about this. Over and over and over again, I find myself on the yoga mat in the same competitive mode, and I'm like, "Oh, it's you again!" to that surface part of myself. So, I try to listen deeper and accept deeper instead of running after physical attainment. There's a bit of svadhyaya (self-study), but also satya (truthfulness) with myself about what yoga is actually about for me.

When she stepped back to reflect on the goals of yoga and the role she wanted it to play in her life, she realized she had a choice. She could practice yoga in a way that made her more available for what matters most in her life, or less available for those things. Like so many bendy yoga practitioners, she had to give up her contortionist tendencies to find a sustainable practice that leaves her ready and able to be who she wants to be in the world.

I want to practice yoga in a way that's not going to be harmful for me in the long term. If I'm not healthy and able to move around and live my life off the yoga mat, then I'm doing a disservice to my family and my kids and the world around me because I can't be of service to others.

Nichi Linder shared some similar thoughts with me during a recent conversation we had. Specifically, the broader perspective facilitated by her yoga and meditation practice has changed her relationship with her physical challenges. It's helped her focus on the most meaningful and purposeful aspects of her life.

Yoga offers a spiritual aspect that can be helpful because the whole point of it is alleviating suffering. Part of that involves being the observer of your own experience—being able to step back and get some perspective on what is going on physically and emotionally so you can separate your being from that. When you take a little bit of a step back, you can start to see that there's more to life than your condition. You get a more nuanced perspective on your experience.

Accepting and nourishing oneself through yoga practice is much different from coming to the yoga mat on an endless quest to fix or perfect something we perceive as inherently flawed. This may have even more relevance for those living with chronic health conditions, in which it can be easy to get stuck wishing things were different rather than accepting things as they are.

In my conversation with Kristine Kaoverii Weber, she emphasized the potential for the inner study of yoga practice to lead to an empowering shift in self-concept.

When you use the practices to get to know yourself better, you can start to reframe the pain, discomfort and frustration that often accompanies chronic health conditions. Yoga can help you start to see yourself and the purpose of your life with more clarity, and understand that you're not your disease.

Incorporating meditation practices that cultivate this type of perspective can enrich your practice and that of your students if you're a teacher. Inviting yourself or your students to reflect on what matters most in life, or to consider a particular yama or niyama is a simple way to invite a shift in perspective. I encourage you to consider the benefits of the whole of the yoga system—ethics, asana, pranayama, and meditation. They can all bring greater ease, more comfort, more understanding, and more acceptance as we navigate life's challenges.

PART 4:

CONCLUSION

CHAPTER 17:

Gathering the Threads

"Yoga offers tools to help shift our perspective about our condition, see ourselves in a different light, and change the story about what's possible."

To build a yoga practice that genuinely supports bendy practitioners, we need to understand yoga, and we need to understand bendiness. Then, we can apply the tools of yoga *appropriately* for bendy people. With this understanding, we can create a practice routine that doesn't contribute to their pain and injury but instead supports their unique needs and makes life better.

In the first chapter of this book, "What is Yoga?", I gave a brief overview of some overarching themes in the yoga tradition. I summarized the eight limbs of yoga presented in the *Yoga Sutras of Patanjali* as a framework to appreciate the variety of tools yoga offers. Yoga invites us on a progressively inward path that leads, in the end, to self-knowledge, self-understanding, and freedom.

Through this book, we've reflected on everything from the ultimate goals of yoga to the behavior of collagen-producing cells, motor control, and many subjects in between. I've presented elements of yoga practice that I find most helpful for bendy people, including specific approaches to asana, pranayama, meditation, and more.

How you put it all together will depend on your interests and your goals. Remember, yoga isn't about the practice. It's about the practitioner. First and foremost, we need a clear intention about why we are practicing yoga and what we hope to gain from it.

Once the intention is clear, we can mix together the "ingredients" of yoga practice in any number of ways to create an enriching experience that supports those intentions. We can include asana, pranayama, mantra, concentration, meditation, relaxation practices, and self-reflection in any practice.

Some questions to guide your reflection about why and how you practice yoga include:

- How can I use asana to cultivate the awareness, boundaries, and stability that will serve me in my life?
- How can I use pranayama to cultivate greater physiological harmony and regulation?
- How can I use meditative practices to learn how to pay attention so I can see myself more clearly?

- How can I use ethical practices to align my behaviors with my values to live according to my purpose?
- How can my yoga practice prepare me to show up fully for what matters most in my life?

I recently had the pleasure of talking with Marlysa Sullivan—yoga therapist, physical therapist, author of *Understanding Yoga Therapy*, and a co-author of *Yoga and Science in Pain Care*—about the unique journey yoga is for each individual. We talked about yoga's potential to bring us closer to our purpose, or dharma. She reflected:

> As we get connected into our body, we get to explore the way we move our body and hold our posture. We get to notice the emotions, the thoughts, the beliefs, and how they're held. For every person it is different. I love the idea of dharma as finding a way of living in harmony with ourselves and the world around us. For someone with hypermobility, the question is: "What type of practice cultivates the qualities they need to find that harmony within themselves?"

For many years I didn't have the right ingredients in my yoga practice. It wasn't helping me cultivate harmony. Instead, it was just the opposite. It had become a performance, driven by what I thought it should look like from the outside. I was in pain every day, and my practice always made it worse.

When I let go of my old ways, my practice became about *me*. My asana practice supported the needs of my body, finally. More importantly, a whole new world opened, and I realized yoga could prepare me for what matters most in my life.

Improving stability and motor control is great (especially for bendy people), but the transformative value of yoga comes from what you learn about yourself in the process. After all, that's what will impact how you show up for the people in your life and how you communicate your boundaries and needs in relationships.

Your practice is *for you*. You get to set your own goals according to your unique needs. Those goals get to change as your needs change over time. Adjust your yoga practice ingredients to support what matters most in your life at any given time.

Your yoga mat (or chair, or whatever surface you use) doesn't have to be a place to work harder, be better, or become different. It can be where you get curious, make your way home to your body, learn about yourself, and transform your experience. It can be a place of anchoring inward to find greater acceptance, comfort, connection, and clarity of purpose. Ultimately, it can be a place for freedom.

Living with a chronic health condition is hard. Sometimes, it can be downright despairing. Yoga won't fix your bendiness or anything else, for that matter. But yoga offers tools to optimize the body and nervous system, manage discomfort, and help us find some perspective and even harmony. Best of all, yoga offers tools to help shift our perspective about our condition, see ourselves in a different light, and change the story about what's possible. It's like putting on a different pair of glasses.

I used to give my yoga teacher trainees a set of heart-shaped glasses made of paper. I'd ask them to decorate the outside with colors, words, or images that reminded them of how they'd like to see others. I'd ask them to do the same on the inside surface to remind them of how they'd like to see themselves. We would all put them on from time to time, especially when we needed a reminder to gaze with curiosity, interest, and love—not just outward, but inward too.

We have a choice about how we make sense of our life circumstances. We can choose to see limitation, or we can choose to see possibility.

If you are a yoga teacher, I hope this book leaves you confident in your understanding of hypermobility syndromes and infused with a new appreciation of the many ways yoga can support bendy people. You are well-equipped to facilitate an enriching yoga experience for your bendy students (and others).

If you are a practitioner, I hope this book leaves you inspired about how yoga can support your best life—from structural integrity, to improved sensory awareness, to nervous system regulation, to deep acceptance of and connection to yourself and the world around you. I hope you feel confident in your ability to make wise modifications to your yoga practice where needed, and excited about how it can celebrate your unique qualities.

If you'd like more practical guidance on practicing or teaching yoga for bendy people, you're in luck. I have developed an on-demand online training with bite-sized lectures and pre-recorded practices to reinforce and further explore concepts and techniques I've discussed in this book. To learn more, visit www.LibbyHinsley.com or www.AnatomyBites. com.

If you're a yoga teacher looking for more anatomy training that's embodied and highly relevant to teaching yoga, visit www.AnatomyBites.com to learn about (and join!) my monthly anatomy membership program.

Acknowledgements

So many people have made this book possible, starting with my parents, Kelley and Sylvia Hinsley, and my big sis, Amy Hinsley. Thank you for cheering me on as I continue to make my way along a sometimes weird and winding path.

Thank you to my dear friend, Mado Hesselink, for always having a metaphorical wide-angle lens handy to show me how to dream bigger.

To Lisa Sherman and Will Hamilton, thank you for your genius, inspiration, support, and for planting the seeds for this book.

To all my teachers, mentors, students, and patients who have taught me about myself, about yoga, about bendiness, and about life: my gratitude is endless.

A special thanks to Emily Nichols Photography for the amazing photographs in this book; and to Miranda Peterson for modeling your bendiness. High-five to Megan Dillon for nailing the book's subtitle.

To all the brave souls who let me interview them for this book and offered their wisdom, insight, or personal stories:

Maria Morrin, Nichi Linder, Sarah Blunkosky, Jules Mitchell, Jill Miller, Judith H. Lasater, Leslie Kaminoff, Kristine Kaoverii Weber, Kate Skinner, Marlysa Sullivan, Lilian Holm, Linda Bluestein, Andrew Beaumont, Kerry Gabrielson, Melanie Downey, Iryna Merideth, Stepfanie Romine, and Trina Altman.

Huge thanks to the people who took the time to read early draft chapters (and in some cases, the entire book!) and offered such thoughtful and thorough feedback. This book is exponentially better for it:

Zorayda Cocchi, Mado Hesselink, Laurie Rush, Teresa Welsch, Kristine Kaoverii Weber, Trina Altman, Jules Mitchell, Jill Miller, Alix Darden, Sascha Frowine, Nina West, Teresa Welsch, Ashley Felkel, DawnMarie Versluys, Bess Park, Stacie Smith, Kachelle Steigerwald, Morgan Davidson, Debbie Phelan, Laura Mahr, Andrew Beaumont, Linda Bluestein, Lisa Sherman, and Will Hamilton.

I am so grateful to all the people who pre-purchased a copy of this book or otherwise supported my presale campaign. Your early support is the only reason this book was able to come to fruition:

Anki Rieger, Jeremy Smith and Chrissie McMullan, Nina West, Angie Ryan, Intan Ridwan, Shvamental Lucy, Liliana Murillo, Tiffany M. Castellanos, John and Bonnie Dings, Isabel Sluitman, Laurel Hicks, Laura M.

Boggess, Valerie Krall, Sam Fox, Jana Franke-Everett, Kathy Newland, Judy Weaver, Christie Martin, Emily Christiansen, Gail Forsyth, Jennifer Tam, Padmaja Reddy, Kelly O'Briant, Peter Elgie, Kate Vickery, Karen McGovern, Stacy Joslin, Laura Tenbrunsel, Jillian Longsworth, Michelle Birmingham, Whitney Yarborough, Megan Dillon, Connie Warden, Jennifer Bouchard, Nicole French, Caitlin Van Hecke, Zorayda Cocchi, Allie Bourgeois, Beth Ashley, Pamela Buckner, Leslie Rhinehart, Natalie Pannemann, Cynthia Lee, Claire Neidecker, Jennifer Rogers, Lauren Flynn, Kathryn Ewing, Iz Webb, Mary Anne Anderson, Janette Wilson, Becca Lee, Erin McCall, Thelma Hinton, Brian Dunn, Michelle Isaacson, Jessica Cleary, Damon Rouse, Jessan Hager, Michelle Martin, Angela Hilton-Prillhart, Teri Dobson, Carrie Klaus, Kristin Peppel, Melinda Travis, Tricia Lea, Ruth Pike-Elliot, Kris Moon, Dana Fehsenfeld, Renee Balyoz, Christopher Fielden, Janis Cronin, Laura Bjorkholm, Lisa Sherman, Beth Tomlinson, Julie Griffis, JoAnn Letten, Melissa Crook, Linette Halcomb, Katherine Hay, Lori Theriault, Caitlyn Phelps, Deirdre Smith-Gilmer, Micah Sexton, Janette Hill, Belinda Brown, Laura Mahr, Corina Stoicescu, Noel Sansotta, Jess Edelstein, Kay McElroy, Libbi Gramling, Alice Kexel, Anna Easterling, Ruth Morrow, Elizabeth Bailey, Barbara Rotondo, Ethel Rhodes, Tanya Kanczuzewski, Andrew Beaumont, Tara Adams, Will Saltz, Sae Smyrl, Robyn Raines, Sarah Filzen, Mary Barnes, Kathryn Ewing, Crystal Harris Chaplick, Amy Bruce, Cat Matlock, Caitlin Brown, Alix Darden, John and Kimberley Puryear, Stephanie Metzger, DawnMarie Versluys, Martha Frierson, Jay Jessee, Cea Rubin, Ellen Crider, Joette Greenway, Amy Rossi, Kelley Hinsley, Renee Brown, Michael Johnson, Erin Marie Porter, Laura Kalthoff, Roxanne

Lenzo, Katie Hall, Marion Stone, Nanci Kaczegowicz, Tami Musumeci-Szabo, Debbie Phelan, Maro Stephenson, Rosemary Mulford, Lisa Isenhart, Deirdre McAdams, Amy Hinsley, Eric Koester, Nila Tiwari Holcombe, Alethea Schaffer, Rosalind Tyburski, Miranda Peterson, Alisha Wielfaert, Rosemary Holbrook, Shala Worsley, Reiko Ando, Denise Johnson, Alix Refshauge, Rosemary Workman, Nancy Brower, Brenda Nakdimen, Laura DeMent, Kirsten Mercer, Terrie Thoma, Aurora Held-Dodd, Cynthia Allen, Emily Dings, Jacqueline Smith, Kristine Weber, Paige Gilchrist, Amy Zellmer, Courtney Brooke Wyatt, Clorinda Roache, Rachel Haley-Katz, and Lily Ackerly.

To Eric Koester and everyone at the Creator Institute and New Degree Press: the work you do in community-powered writing and publishing is inspiring, and I'm so grateful to be part of it. A special thanks to my editors, Benay Stein and Stephanie McKibben, who have held my hand through this entire process and could see where I was going even when I couldn't.

And so many more. Every kindness and every word of encouragement along the way has been everything.

Appendix

INTRODUCTION

Demmler, Joanne C., Mark D. Atkinson, Emma J. Reinhold, Ernest Choy, Ronan A. Lyons, and Sinead T. Brophy. "Diagnosed Prevalence of Ehlers-Danlos Syndrome and Hypermobility Spectrum Disorder in Wales, UK: A National Electronic Cohort Study and Case–Control Comparison." *BMJ Open* 9, no. 11 (2019): e031365. https://doi.org/10.1136/bmjopen-2019-031365.

Krishnamacharya Yoga Mandiram. "About KYM, Chennai's Most Authentic and Traditional Yoga Centre." Krishnamacharya Yoga Mandiram. 2019. December 30, 2021. http://www.kym.org/about-kym/.

CHAPTER 1: WHAT IS YOGA?

Desikachar, T.K.V. The Heart of Yoga. Rochester, VT: Inner Traditions International Press, 1999.

Desikachar, T.K.V. *Reflections on Yoga Sutras of Patanjali.* Nandanam, Chennai: Quadra Press Ltd, 2008.

Feuerstein, Georg. *The Yoga Tradition*. Prescott, AZ: Hohm Press, 1998.

Gard, Tim, Jessica J. Noggle, Crystal L. Park, David R. Vago, and Angela Wilson. "Potential Self-Regulatory Mechanisms of Yoga for Psychological Health." *Frontiers in Human Neuroscience* 8 (2014): 770. https://doi.org/10.3389/fnhum.2014.00770.

Nhat Hanh, Thich, and Mobi Ho. *Old Path, White Clouds: Walking in the Footsteps of the Buddha*. Berkeley, Calif: Parallax Press, 1991.

Yoga Alliance. "2016 Yoga in America Study." Yoga Alliance. 2021. Accessed December 31, 2021. https://www.yogaalliance. org/2016yogainamericastudy.

CHAPTER 2: HYPERMOBILITY 101

Atwell, Karina, William Michael, Jared Dubey, Sarah James, Andrea Martonffy, Scott Anderson, Nathan Rudin, and Sarina Schrager. "Diagnosis and Management of Hypermobility Spectrum Disorders in Primary Care." *The Journal of the American Board of Family Medicine* 34, no. 4 (2021): 838–48. https://doi. org/10.3122/jabfm.2021.04.200374.

Aubry-Rozier, Bérengère, Adrien Schwitzguebel, Flore Valerio, Joelle Tanniger, Célia Paquier, Chantal Berna, Thomas Hügle, and Charles Benaim. "Are Patients with Hypermobile Ehlers-Danlos Syndrome or Hypermobility Spectrum Disorder so Different?" *Rheumatology International* 41, no. 10 (2021): 1785–94. https://doi.org/10.1007/s00296-021-04968-3.

Bockhorn, Lauren N., Angelina M. Vera, David Dong, Domenica A. Delgado, Kevin E. Varner, and Joshua D. Harris. "Interrater and Intrarater Reliability of the Beighton Score: A Systematic Review." *Orthopaedic Journal of Sports Medicine* 9, no. 1 (January 1, 2021): 232596712096809. https://doi.org/10.1177/2325967120968099.

Bowen, Jessica M., Glenda J. Sobey, Nigel P. Burrows, Marina Colombi, Mark E. Lavallee, Fransiska Malfait, and Clair A. Francomano. "Ehlers-Danlos Syndrome, Classical Type." *American Journal of Medical Genetics Part C: Seminars in Medical Genetics* 175, no. 1 (2017): 27–39. https://doi.org/10.1002/ajmg.c.31548.

Byers, Peter H., John Belmont, James Black, Julie De Backer, Michael Frank, Xavier Jeunemaitre, Diana Johnson, et al. "Diagnosis, Natural History, and Management in Vascular Ehlers-Danlos Syndrome." *American Journal of Medical Genetics Part C: Seminars in Medical Genetics* 175, no. 1 (2017): 40–47. https://doi.org/10.1002/ajmg.c.31553.

Castori, Marco, Brad Tinkle, Howard Levy, Rodney Grahame, Fransiska Malfait, and Alan Hakim. "A Framework for the Classification of Joint Hypermobility and Related Conditions." *American Journal of Medical Genetics Part C: Seminars in Medical Genetics* 175, no. 1 (2017): 148–57. https://doi.org/10.1002/ajmg.c.31539.

Cleveland Clinic. "POTS: Causes, Symptoms, Diagnosis, & Treatment." Cleveland Clinic. 2021. December 31, 2021. https://my.clevelandclinic.org/health/diseases/16560-postural-orthostatic-tachycardia-syndrome-pots.

Davis, Shirley. "Medical and Mental Health Gaslighting and Iatrogenic Injury." CPTSD Foundation. 2020. Accessed February 20, 2022. https://cptsdfoundation.org/2020/06/08/medical-and-mental-health-gaslighting-and-iatrogenic-injury/.

Demmler, Joanne C., Mark D. Atkinson, Emma J. Reinhold, Ernest Choy, Ronan A. Lyons, and Sinead T. Brophy. "Diagnosed Prevalence of Ehlers-Danlos Syndrome and Hypermobility Spectrum Disorder in Wales, UK: A National Electronic Cohort Study and Case–Control Comparison." *BMJ Open* 9, no. 11 (2019): e031365. https://doi.org/10.1136/bmjopen-2019-031365.

Glans, Martin, Mats B. Humble, Marie Elwin, and Susanne Bejerot. "Self-Rated Joint Hypermobility: The Five-Part Questionnaire Evaluated in a Swedish Non-Clinical Adult Population." *BMC Musculoskeletal Disorders* 21, no. 1 (2020): 174. https://doi.org/10.1186/s12891-020-3067-1.

Magee, David J. *Orthopedic Physical Assessment.* St. Louis, MO: Saunders Elsevier Press, 2008.

Malek, Sabeeha, and Darius Koster. "The Role of Cell Adhesion and Cytoskeleton Dynamics in the Pathogenesis of the Ehlers-Danlos Syndromes and Hypermobility Spectrum Disorders." *Frontiers in Cell and Developmental Biology* 9 (April 2021): 1-13. https://doi.org/10.3389/fcell.2021.649082.

Meyer, Kaitlin J., Cliffton Chan, Luke Hopper, and Leslie L. Nicholson. "Identifying Lower Limb Specific and Generalised Joint Hypermobility in Adults: Validation of the Lower Limb Assessment Score." *BMC Musculoskeletal Disorders* 18, no. 1 (2017): 514. https://doi.org/10.1186/s12891-017-1875-8.

Nicholson, Leslie L., and Cliffton Chan. "The Upper Limb Hypermobility Assessment Tool: A Novel Validated Measure of Adult Joint Mobility." *Musculoskeletal Science and Practice* 35 (2018): 38–45. https://doi.org/10.1016/j.msksp.2018.02.006.

Parapia, Liakat, and Carolyn Jackson. "Ehlers-Danlos Syndrome–A Historical Review." *British Journal of Haematology* 141, no. 1 (March 2008): 32-35. https://doi.org/10.1111/j.1365-2141.2008.06994.x.

Ramcharan, Michael, and Lyndsay Andrews. "Clinical Brief: Recognition of Benign Joint Hypermobility Syndrome (BJHS)." *Topics in Integrative Health Care* 3, no. 1 (March 2012) ID: 3.1005 http://www.tihcij.com/Articles/Clinical-Brief-Recognition-of-Benign-Joint-Hypermobility-Syndrome-BJHS.aspx-?id=0000345.

Simpson, Michael R. "Benign Joint Hypermobility Syndrome: Evaluation, Diagnosis, and Management." *The Journal of the American Osteopathic Association* 106, no. 9 (September 2006): 531–36.

The Ehlers-Danlos Society. "EDS Types." The Ehlers-Danlos Society. 2021. Accessed December 20, 2021. https://www.ehlers-danlos.com/eds-types/.

The Ehlers-Danlos Society. "hEDS Diagnostic Checklist." The Ehlers-Danlos Society. 2021. Accessed December 30, 2021. https://www.ehlers-danlos.com/heds-diagnostic-checklist/.

The Ehlers-Danlos Society. "What are the Ehlers-Danlos Syndromes?" The Ehlers-Danlos Society. 2021. Accessed December 30, 2021. https://www.ehlers-danlos.com/what-is-eds/.

The Ehlers-Danlos Society. "Why the zebra?" The Ehlers-Danlos Society. 2021. Accessed December 30, 2021. https://www.ehlers-danlos.com/why-the-zebra/.

Voermans, Nicol C., Hans Knoop, Gijs Bleijenberg, and Baziel G. van Engelen. "Pain in Ehlers-Danlos Syndrome Is Common, Severe, and Associated with Functional Impairment." *Journal of Pain and Symptom Management* 40, no. 3 (2010): 370–78. https://doi.org/10.1016/j.jpainsymman.2009.12.026.

CHAPTER 3: CONNECTIVE TISSUE NITTY-GRITTY

Abboud, Jacques, François Nougarou, and Martin Descarreaux. "Muscle Activity Adaptations to Spinal Tissue Creep in the Presence of Muscle Fatigue." Edited by Francesco Cappello. *PLOS ONE* 11, no. 2 (February 11, 2016): e0149076. https://doi.org/10.1371/journal.pone.0149076.

Alsiri, Najla, Saud Al-Obaidi, Akram Asbeutah, Mariam Almandeel, and Shea Palmer. "The Impact of Hypermobility Spectrum Disorders on Musculoskeletal Tissue Stiffness: An Exploration Using Strain Elastography." *Clinical Rheumatology* 38, no. 1 (2019): 85–95. https://doi.org/10.1007/s10067-018-4193-0.

Arseni, Lavinia, Anita Lombardi, and Donata Orioli. "From Structure to Phenotype: Impact of Collagen Alterations on Human Health." *International Journal of Molecular Sciences* 19, no. 5 (May 8, 2018): 1407. https://doi.org/10.3390/ijms19051407.

Cyron, C. J., and J. D. Humphrey. "Growth and Remodeling of Load-Bearing Biological Soft Tissues." *Meccanica* 52, no. 3 (2017): 645–64. https://doi.org/10.1007/s11012-016-0472-5.

Ergen, Emin, and Bülent Ulkar. "Proprioception and Coordination." In *Clinical Sports Medicine*, 237–55. Elsevier, 2007. https://doi.org/10.1016/B978-141602443-9.50021-0.

Iheanacho, Franklin, and Anantha Ramana Vellipuram. "Physiology, Mechanoreceptors." In *StatPearls*. Treasure Island (FL): StatPearls Publishing, 2021. http://www.ncbi.nlm.nih.gov/books/NBK541068/.

Kamrani, Payvand, Geoffrey Marston, and Arif Jan. "Anatomy, Connective Tissue." In *StatPearls*. Treasure Island (FL): StatPearls Publishing, 2021. http://www.ncbi.nlm.nih.gov/books/NBK538534/.

Kendall, Ryan T., and Carol A. Feghali-Bostwick. "Fibroblasts in Fibrosis: Novel Roles and Mediators." *Frontiers in Pharmacology* 5 (May 27, 2014). https://doi.org/10.3389/fphar.2014.00123.

Kumka, Myroslava, and Jason Bonar. "Fascia: a morphological description and classification system based on a literature review." *The Journal of the Canadian Chiropractic Association* vol. 56,3 (2012): 179-91.

Mitchell, Jules. *Yoga Biomechanics: Stretching Redefined*. Pencaitland, UK: Handspring Publishing Limited, 2019.

Møller, Mathias Bech, Michael Kjær, René Brüggebusch Svensson, Jesper Lovind Andersen, Stig Peter Magnusson, and Rie Harboe Nielsen. "Functional Adaptation of Tendon and Skeletal Muscle to Resistance Training in Three Patients with Genetically Verified Classic Ehlers-Danlos Syndrome." *Muscles, Ligaments and Tendons Journal* 4, no. 3 (July 2014): 315–23.

Palmer, Shea, Elise Denner, Matthew Riglar, Holly Scannell, Sarah Webb, and Georgina Young. "Quantitative Measures of Tissue Mechanics to Detect Hypermobile Ehlers-Danlos Syndrome and Hypermobility Syndrome Disorders: A Systematic Review." *Clinical Rheumatology* 39, no. 3 (2020): 715–25. https://doi.org/10.1007/s10067-020-04939-2.

Panjabi, Manohar M. "The Stabilizing System of the Spine. Part I. Function, Dysfunction, Adaptation, and Enhancement:" *Journal of Spinal Disorders* 5, no. 4 (1992): 383–89. https://doi.org/10.1097/00002517-199212000-00001.

Provenzano, Paolo P., and Ray Vanderby. "Collagen Fibril Morphology and Organization: Implications for Force Transmission in Ligament and Tendon." *Matrix Biology* 25, no. 2 (2006): 71–84. https://doi.org/10.1016/j.matbio.2005.09.005.

Purslow, Peter, and Jean-Paul Delage. "General anatomy of the muscle fasciae." In *Fascia: The Tensional Network of the Human Body,* edited By Robert Schleip, Thomas W. Findley, Leon Chaitow, and Peter A. Huijing, 6-10. Amsterdam, Netherlands: Elsevier, 2012.

Rombaut, Lies, Fransiska Malfait, Inge De Wandele, Nele Mahieu, Youri Thijs, Patrick Segers, Anne De Paepe, and Patrick Calders. "Muscle-Tendon Tissue Properties in the Hypermobility Type of Ehlers-Danlos Syndrome: Muscle Tension and Achilles Tendon Stiffness in EDS-HT Patients." *Arthritis Care & Research* 64, no. 5 (2012): 766–72. https://doi.org/10.1002/acr.21592.

Schleip, Robert, Heike Jager, and Werner Klingler. "Fascia Is Alive." In *Fascia: The Tensional Network of the Human Body,* edited By Robert Schleip, Thomas W. Findley, Leon Chaitow, and Peter A. Huijing, 157–164. Amsterdam, Netherlands: Elsevier, 2012.

Shanb, Alsayed A., and Enas F. Youssef. "The Impact of Adding Weight-Bearing Exercise Versus Nonweight Bearing Programs to the Medical Treatment of Elderly Patients with Osteoporosis." *Journal of Family and Community Medicine* 21, no. 3 (2014): 176. https://doi.org/10.4103/2230-8229.142972.

Stecco, Carla. *Functional Atlas of the Human Fascial System.* Amsterdam, Netherlands: Elsevier, 2015.

Willard, Frank H. "Somatic fascia." In *Fascia: The Tensional Network of the Human Body,* edited By Robert Schleip, Thomas W. Findley, Leon Chaitow, and Peter A. Huijing, 11–17. Amsterdam, Netherlands: Elsevier, 2012.

Zitnay, Jared L., and Jeffrey A. Weiss. "Load Transfer, Damage, and Failure in Ligaments and Tendons." *Journal of Orthopaedic Research®* 36, no. 12 (2018): 3093–3104. https://doi.org/10.1002/jor.24134.

CHAPTER 4: COMMON BENDY BODY COMPLAINTS

Ali, Ahmed, Paul Andrzejowski, Nikolaos K. Kanakaris, and Peter V. Giannoudis. "Pelvic Girdle Pain, Hypermobility Spectrum Disorder and Hypermobility-Type Ehlers-Danlos Syndrome: A

Narrative Literature Review." *Journal of Clinical Medicine* 9, no. 12 (December 9, 2020): 3992. https://doi.org/10.3390/jcm9123992.

Baeza-Velasco, Carolina, Maude Seneque, Philippe Courtet, Émilie Olié, Charles Chatenet, Paola Espinoza, Geraldine Dorard, and Sébastien Guillaume. "Joint Hypermobility and Clinical Correlates in a Group of Patients with Eating Disorders." *Frontiers in Psychiatry* (January 12, 2022): 2485. https://doi.org/10.3389/fpsyt.2021.803614.

Beijk, Iris, Rob Knoef, Arie van Vugt, Wiebe Verra, and Jorm Nellensteijn. "Sacroiliac Joint Fusion in Patients with Ehlers-Danlos Syndrome: A Case Series." *North American Spine Society Journal (NASSJ)* 8 (2021): 100082. https://doi.org/10.1016/j.xnsj.2021.100082.

Boomershine, Chad S. "Fibromyalgia: The Prototypical Central Sensitivity Syndrome." *Current Rheumatology Reviews* 11, no. 2 (2015): 131–45. https://doi.org/10.2174/1573397111666150619095007.

Bulbena, Antoni, Joan C. Duró, Miguel Porta, Rocío Martín-Santos, Antonio Mateo, Lluis Molina, Ramon Vallescar, and Julio Vallejo. "Anxiety Disorders in the Joint Hypermobility Syndrome." *Psychiatry Research* 46, no. 1 (1993): 59–68. https://doi.org/10.1016/0165-1781(93)90008-5.

Casanova, Emily L., Carolina Baeza-Velasco, Caroline B. Buchanan, and Manuel F. Casanova. "The Relationship between Autism and Ehlers-Danlos Syndromes/Hypermobility Spectrum Disorders." *Journal of Personalized Medicine* 10, no. 4 (December 1, 2020): 260. https://doi.org/10.3390/jpm10040260.

Clayton, Holly A, Stephanie A H Jones, and Denise Y P Henriques. "Proprioceptive Precision Is Impaired in Ehlers-Danlos Syndrome." *SpringerPlus* 4, no. 1 (2015): 323. https://doi.org/10.1186/s40064-015-1089-1.

Cleveland Clinic. "POTS (Postural Orthostatic Tachycardia Syndrome) and Chronic Pain." Cleveland Clinic. 2022. Accessed February 16, 2022. https://my.clevelandclinic.org/health/articles/21124-postural-orthostatic-tachycardia-syndrome-pots-and-chronic-pain.

Csecs, Jenny L L, Valeria Iodice, Charlotte L Rae, Alice Brooke, Rebecca Simmons, Nicholas G Dowell, Fenella Prowse, Kristy Themelis, Hugo D Critchley, and Jessica A Eccles. "Increased Rate of Joint Hypermobility in Autism and Related Neurodevelopmental Conditions Is Linked to Dysautonomia and Pain." Preprint. *Psychiatry and Clinical Psychology*, September 15, 2020. https://doi.org/10.1101/2020.09.14.20194118.

Cutts, R.M., R. Meyer, N. Thapar, K. Rigby, C. Schwarz, S. Mailliard, and N. Shah. "Gastrointestinal Food Allergies in Children with Ehlers-Danlos Type 3 Syndrome." *Journal of Allergy and Clinical Immunology* 129, no. 2 (2012): AB34. https://doi.org/10.1016/j.jaci.2011.12.789.

Cutts, Steven, Mark Prempeh, and Steven Drew. "Anterior Shoulder Dislocation." *The Annals of The Royal College of Surgeons of England* 91, no. 1 (2009): 2–7. https://doi.org/10.1308/003588409X359123.

Eccles, Jessica A., Beth Thompson, Kristy Themelis, Marisa L. Amato, Robyn Stocks, Amy Pound, Anna-Marie Jones, et al.

"Beyond Bones: The Relevance of Variants of Connective Tissue (Hypermobility) to Fibromyalgia, ME/CFS and Controversies Surrounding Diagnostic Classification: An Observational Study." *Clinical Medicine* 21, no. 1 (2021): 53–58. https://doi.org/10.7861/clinmed.2020-0743.

Eccles, Jessica A., F. D. C. Beacher, M. A. Gray, C. L. Jones, L. Minati, N. A. Harrison, and H. D. Critchley. "Brain Structure and Joint Hypermobility: Relevance to the Expression of Psychiatric Symptoms." *British Journal of Psychiatry* 200, no. 6 (2012): 508–9. https://doi.org/10.1192/bjp.bp.111.092460.

Eccles, J., V. Iodice, N. Dowell, A. Owens, L. Hughes, S. Skipper, Y. Lycette, et al. "Joint Hypermobility and Autonomic Hyperactivity: Relevance to Neurodevelopmental Disorders." *Journal of Neurology, Neurosurgery & Psychiatry* 85, no. 8 (August 1, 2014): e3–e3. https://doi.org/10.1136/jnnp-2014-308883.9.

Eccles, Jessica, Andrew Owens, Neil Harrison, Rodney Grahame, and Hugo Critchley. "Joint Hypermobility and Autonomic Hyperactivity: An Autonomic and Functional Neuroimaging Study." *The Lancet* 387 (2016): S40. https://doi.org/10.1016/S0140-6736(16)00427-X.

Fikree, Asma, Gisela Chelimsky, Heidi Collins, Katcha Kovacic, and Qasim Aziz. "Gastrointestinal Involvement in the Ehlers-Danlos Syndromes." *American Journal of Medical Genetics Part C: Seminars in Medical Genetics* 175, no. 1 (2017): 181–87. https://doi.org/10.1002/ajmg.c.31546.

Gazit, Yael, A. Menahem Nahir, Rodney Grahame, and Giris Jacob. "Dysautonomia in the Joint Hypermobility Syndrome." *The*

American Journal of Medicine 115, no. 1 (2003): 33–40. https://
doi.org/10.1016/S0002-9343(03)00235-3.

Gilliam, Elizabeth, Jodi D. Hoffman, and Gloria Yeh. "Urogenital
and Pelvic Complications in the Ehlers-Danlos Syndromes
and Associated Hypermobility Spectrum Disorders: A Scoping
Review." *Clinical Genetics* 97, no. 1 (2020): 168–78. https://doi.
org/10.1111/cge.13624.

Glans, Martin, Nils Thelin, Mats B. Humble, Marie Elwin, and
Susanne Bejerot. "Association between Adult Attention-Deficit
Hyperactivity Disorder and Generalised Joint Hypermobility:
A Cross-Sectional Case Control Comparison." *Journal of Psy-
chiatric Research* 143 (2021): 334–40. https://doi.org/10.1016/j.
jpsychires.2021.07.006.

Goh, Min, James Olver, Chia Huang, Melinda Millard, and Chris
O'Callaghan. "Prevalence and Familial Patterns of Gastroin-
testinal Symptoms, Joint Hypermobility and Diurnal Blood
Pressure Variations in Patients with Anorexia Nervosa."
Journal of Eating Disorders 1, no. S1 (2013): O45. https://doi.
org/10.1186/2050-2974-1-S1-O45.

Groh, Megan M., and Joseph Herrera. "A Comprehensive Review
of Hip Labral Tears." *Current Reviews in Musculoskeletal Medicine* 2, no. 2 (2009): 105–17. https://doi.org/10.1007/s12178-009-
9052-9.

Hakim, Alan, Inge De Wandele, Chris O'Callaghan, Alan Pocinki,
and Peter Rowe. "Chronic Fatigue in Ehlers-Danlos Syn-
drome-Hypermobile Type." *American Journal of Medical*

Genetics Part C: Seminars in Medical Genetics 175, no. 1 (2017): 175–80. https://doi.org/10.1002/ajmg.c.31542.

Hicks, Allen. "What Is the Difference Between Tendinitis, Tendinosis, and Tendinopathy?" Evolution Physiotherapy. Accessed January 2, 2022. https://evolutionphysiotherapy.com/what-is-the-difference-between-tendinitis-tendinosis-and-tendinopathy-at-evolution-physiotherapy-2/.

Hugon-Rodin, Justine, Géraldine Lebègue, Stéphanie Becourt, Claude Hamonet, and Anne Gompel. "Gynecologic Symptoms and the Influence on Reproductive Life in 386 Women with Hypermobility Type Ehlers-Danlos Syndrome: A Cohort Study." *Orphanet Journal of Rare Diseases* 11, no. 1 (2016): 124. https://doi.org/10.1186/s13023-016-0511-2.

Jacquemot, Aimée Margarita Marisol Catherine, and Rebecca Park. "The Role of Interoception in the Pathogenesis and Treatment of Anorexia Nervosa: A Narrative Review." *Frontiers in Psychiatry* 11 (April 17, 2020): 281. https://doi.org/10.3389/fpsyt.2020.00281.

Kavuncu, Vural, Sezai Sahin, Ayhan Kamanli, Ayse Karan, and Cihan Aksoy. "The Role of Systemic Hypermobility and Condylar Hypermobility in Temporomandibular Joint Dysfunction Syndrome." *Rheumatology International* 26, no. 3 (2006): 257–60. https://doi.org/10.1007/s00296-005-0620-z.

Khurana, Ramesh K. "Coat-Hanger Ache in Orthostatic Hypotension." *Cephalalgia* 32, no. 10 (2012): 731–37. https://doi.org/10.1177/0333102412449932.

Kohn, Alison, and Christopher Chang. "The Relationship Between Hypermobile Ehlers-Danlos Syndrome (HEDS), Postural Orthostatic Tachycardia Syndrome (POTS), and Mast Cell Activation Syndrome (MCAS)." *Clinical Reviews in Allergy & Immunology* 58, no. 3 (2020): 273–97. https://doi.org/10.1007/s12016-019-08755-8.

Mack, Kenneth J., Jonathan N. Johnson, and Peter C. Rowe. "Orthostatic Intolerance and the Headache Patient." *Seminars in Pediatric Neurology* 17, no. 2 (2010): 109–16. https://doi.org/10.1016/j.spen.2010.04.006.

Magee, David J. *Orthopedic Physical Assessment.* St. Louis, MO: Saunders Elsevier Press, 2008.

Makol, A.K., B. Chakravorty, M.B. Heller, and B. Riley. "The Association Between Hypermobility Ehlers–Danlos Syndrome and Other Rheumatologic Diseases." *European Medical Journal*, November 8, 2021. https://doi.org/10.33590/emj/21-00078R2.

MallorquÃ-BaguÃ©, NÃoria, Sarah N. Garfinkel, Miriam Engels, Jessica A. Eccles, Guillem Pailhez, Antonio Bulbena, and Hugo D. Critchley. "Neuroimaging and Psychophysiological Investigation of the Link between Anxiety, Enhanced Affective Reactivity and Interoception in People with Joint Hypermobility." *Frontiers in Psychology* 5 (October 14, 2014). https://doi.org/10.3389/fpsyg.2014.01162.

Martín-Santos, Rocío, Antonio Bulbena, Miquel Porta, Jordi Gago, Lluís Molina, and Juan C. Duró. "Association Between Joint Hypermobility Syndrome and Panic Disorder." *Ameri-*

can *Journal of Psychiatry* 155, no. 11 (1998): 1578–83. https://doi.
org/10.1176/ajp.155.11.1578.

Mathias, Christopher J., David A. Low, Valeria Iodice, Andrew P.
Owens, Mojca Kirbis, and Rodney Grahame. "Postural Tachycardia Syndrome—Current Experience and Concepts." *Nature
Reviews Neurology* 8, no. 1 (2012): 22–34. https://doi.org/10.1038/
nrneurol.2011.187.

Maya, Tania Ruiz, Veronica Fettig, Lakshmi Mehta, Bruce D. Gelb,
and Amy R. Kontorovich. "Dysautonomia in Hypermobile
Ehlers-Danlos Syndrome and Hypermobility Spectrum Disorders Is Associated with Exercise Intolerance and Cardiac
Atrophy." Preprint. *Genetic and Genomic Medicine*, February
9, 2021. https://doi.org/10.1101/2021.02.08.21251338.

Milhorat, Thomas H., Paolo A. Bolognese, Misao Nishikawa, Nazli
B. McDonnell, and Clair A. Francomano. "Syndrome of Occip-
itoatlantoaxial Hypermobility, Cranial Settling, and Chiari
Malformation Type I in Patients with Hereditary Disorders
of Connective Tissue." *Journal of Neurosurgery: Spine* 7, no. 6
(December 1, 2007): 601–9. https://doi.org/10.3171/SPI-07/12/601.

Moss, C., J. Fernandez-Mendoza, J. Schubart, T. Sheehan, A. Schil-
ling, C. Francomano, and R. Bascom. "Nighttime Sleep and
Daytime Functioning in Ehlers-Danlos Syndrome: A Cohort
Study of Syndrome Subtypes." *Sleep* 41, no. suppl_1 (April 27,
2018): A343–A343. https://doi.org/10.1093/sleep/zsy061.923.

Muldoon, Michael, Gregory Gosey, Robert Healey, and Richard
Santore. "Hypermobility: A Key Factor in Hip Dysplasia. A
Prospective Evaluation of 266 Patients." *Journal of Hip Pres-*

ervation Surgery 3, no. suppl_1 (2016). https://doi.org/10.1093/jhps/hnw030.034.

National Institute of Neurological Disorders and Stroke. "Chiari Malformation Fact Sheet." National Institute of Neurological Disorders and Stroke. Accessed January 2, 2022. https://www.ninds.nih.gov/Disorders/Patient-Caregiver-Education/Fact-Sheets/Chiari-Malformation-Fact-Sheet.

Umeda, Satoshi, Neil A. Harrison, Marcus A. Gray, Christopher J. Mathias, and Hugo D. Critchley. "Structural Brain Abnormalities in Postural Tachycardia Syndrome: A VBM-DARTEL Study." *Frontiers in Neuroscience* 9 (March 17, 2015). https://doi.org/10.3389/fnins.2015.00034.

Mayo Foundation for Medical Education and Research. "Chronic Fatigue Syndrome—Symptoms and Causes." Mayo Foundation for Medical Education and Research. Accessed January 2, 2022. https://www.mayoclinic.org/diseases-conditions/chronic-fatigue-syndrome/symptoms-causes/syc-20360490.

Piech, Richard M., Daniela Strelchuk, Jake Knights, Jonathan V. Hjälmheden, Jonas K. Olofsson, and Jane E. Aspell. "People with Higher Interoceptive Sensitivity Are More Altruistic, but Improving Interoception Does Not Increase Altruism." *Scientific Reports* 7, no. 1 (2017): 15652. https://doi.org/10.1038/s41598-017-14318-8.

Register, Brad, Andrew T. Pennock, Charles P. Ho, Colin D. Strickland, Ashur Lawand, and Marc J. Philippon. "Prevalence of Abnormal Hip Findings in Asymptomatic Participants: A Prospective, Blinded Study." *The American Journal*

of Sports Medicine 40, no. 12 (2012): 2720–24. https://doi.
org/10.1177/0363546512462124.

Riggs, Kelsey, Lauren Babcock, Vernon Rowe, John Hunter, Doug
Schell, Arlene O'Shea, Dorsey Paul, Gloria Ortiz-Guerrero,
and James Barnett. "Symptoms of Hypermobility Spectrum
Disorder May Mimic Multiple Sclerosis." *Neurology* 90, no. 15
Supplement (April 2018): S44.003.

Rodgers, Kyla R., Jiang Gui, Mary Beth P. Dinulos, and Richard
C. Chou. "Ehlers-Danlos Syndrome Hypermobility Type Is
Associated with Rheumatic Diseases." *Scientific Reports* 7, no.
1 (2017): 39636. https://doi.org/10.1038/srep39636.

Shirley, Eric D., Marlene DeMaio, and Joanne Bodurtha.
"Ehlers-Danlos Syndrome in Orthopaedics: Etiology, Diagnosis, and Treatment Implications." *Sports Health: A Mul-
tidisciplinary Approach* 4, no. 5 (2012): 394–403. https://doi.
org/10.1177/1941738112452385.

Tinkle, Brad T. "Symptomatic Joint Hypermobility." *Best Practice & Research Clinical Rheumatology* 34, no. 3 (2020): 101508.
https://doi.org/10.1016/j.berh.2020.101508.

CHAPTER 7: SMALLER AND SLOWER MOVEMENTS

Doidge, Norman. *The Brain's Way of Healing*. New York, NY:
Viking Press, 2015.

Rassier, D. E., B. R. MacIntosh, and W. Herzog. "Length Depen-
dence of Active Force Production in Skeletal Muscle." *Journal*

of Applied Physiology 86, no. 5 (May 1, 1999): 1445–57. https://doi.org/10.1152/jappl.1999.86.5.1445.

Shumway-Cook A., Woollacott M. *Motor Control: Translating Research into Clinical Practice*. Philadelphia: Lippincott Williams & Wilkins, 2007.

Villemure, Chantal, Marta ÄŒeko, Valerie A. Cotton, and M. Catherine Bushnell. "Neuroprotective Effects of Yoga Practice: Age-, Experience-, and Frequency-Dependent Plasticity." *Frontiers in Human Neuroscience* 9 (May 12, 2015). https://doi.org/10.3389/fnhum.2015.00281.

CHAPTER 8: STRETCHING

Abboud, Jacques, François Nougarou, and Martin Descarreaux. "Muscle Activity Adaptations to Spinal Tissue Creep in the Presence of Muscle Fatigue." Edited by Francesco Cappello. *PLOS ONE* 11, no. 2 (February 11, 2016): e0149076. https://doi.org/10.1371/journal.pone.0149076.

Berrueta, Lisbeth, Igla Muskaj, Sara Olenich, Taylor Butler, Gary J. Badger, Romain A. Colas, Matthew Spite, Charles N. Serhan, and Helene M. Langevin. "Stretching Impacts Inflammation Resolution in Connective Tissue." *Journal of Cellular Physiology* 231, no. 7 (2016): 1621–27. https://doi.org/10.1002/jcp.25263.

Berrueta, L., J. Bergholz, D. Munoz, I. Muskaj, G. J. Badger, A. Shukla, H. J. Kim, J. J. Zhao, and H. M. Langevin. "Stretching Reduces Tumor Growth in a Mouse Breast Cancer Model." *Scientific Reports* 8, no. 1 (2018): 7864. https://doi.org/10.1038/s41598-018-26198-7.

Docking, S., T. Samiric, E. Scase, C. Purdam, and J. Cook. "Relationship between Compressive Loading and ECM Changes in Tendons." *Muscle Ligaments and Tendons Journal* 03, no. 01 (2019): 7. https://doi.org/10.32098/mltj.01.2013.03.

Inami, Takayuki, Takuya Shimizu, Reizo Baba, and Akemi Nakagaki. "Acute Changes in Autonomic Nerve Activity during Passive Static Stretching." *American Journal of Sports Science and Medicine* 2, no. 4 (July 13, 2014): 166–70. https://doi.org/10.12691/ajssm-2-4-9.

Møller, Mathias Bech, Michael Kjær, René Brüggebusch Svensson, Jesper Lovind Andersen, Stig Peter Magnusson, and Rie Harboe Nielsen. "Functional Adaptation of Tendon and Skeletal Muscle to Resistance Training in Three Patients with Genetically Verified Classic Ehlers-Danlos Syndrome." *Muscles, Ligaments and Tendons Journal* 4, no. 3 (July 2014): 315–23.

Montero-Marín, Jesús, Sonia Asún, Nerea Estrada-Marcén, Rosario Romero, and Roberto Asún. "Effectiveness of a Stretching Program on Anxiety Levels of Workers in a Logistic Platform: A Randomized Controlled Study." *Atención Primaria* 45, no. 7 (2013): 376–83. https://doi.org/10.1016/j.aprim.2013.03.002.

Provenzano, Paolo P., and Ray Vanderby. "Collagen Fibril Morphology and Organization: Implications for Force Transmission in Ligament and Tendon." *Matrix Biology* 25, no. 2 (2006): 71–84. https://doi.org/10.1016/j.matbio.2005.09.005.

Rombaut, Lies, Fransiska Malfait, Inge De Wandele, Nele Mahieu, Youri Thijs, Patrick Segers, Anne De Paepe, and Patrick Calders. "Muscle-Tendon Tissue Properties in the Hypermobility Type of Ehlers-Danlos Syndrome: Muscle Tension and Achilles Tendon Stiffness in EDS-HT Patients." *Arthritis Care & Research* 64, no. 5 (2012): 766–72. https://doi.org/10.1002/acr.21592.

Rowlands, Ann V., Vicky F. Marginson, and Jonathan Lee. "Chronic Flexibility Gains: Effect of Isometric Contraction Duration during Proprioceptive Neuromuscular Facilitation Stretching Techniques." *Research Quarterly for Exercise and Sport* 74, no. 1 (2003): 47–51. https://doi.org/10.1080/02701367.2003.10609063.

Stecco, Carla. *Functional Atlas of the Human Fascial System.* Amsterdam, Netherlands: Elsevier, 2015.

Tworoger, Shelley S., Yutaka Yasui, Michael V. Vitiello, Robert S. Schwartz, Cornelia M. Ulrich, Erin J. Aiello, Melinda L. Irwin, Deborah Bowen, John D. Potter, and Anne McTiernan. "Effects of a Yearlong Moderate-Intensity Exercise and a Stretching Intervention on Sleep Quality in Postmenopausal Women." *Sleep* 26, no. 7 (2003): 830–36. https://doi.org/10.1093/sleep/26.7.830.

Zitnay, Jared L., and Jeffrey A. Weiss. "Load Transfer, Damage, and Failure in Ligaments and Tendons." *Journal of Orthopaedic Research®* 36, no. 12 (2018): 3093–3104. https://doi.org/10.1002/jor.24134.

CHAPTER 9: STRENGTH AND STABILITY

Coussens, Marie, Patrick Calders, Bruno Lapauw, Bert Celie, Thiberiu Banica, Inge De Wandele, Verity Pacey, Fransis Malfait, and Lies Rombaut. "Does Muscle Strength Change Over

Time in Patients With Hypermobile Ehlers-Danlos Syndrome/
Hypermobility Spectrum Disorder? An Eight-Year Follow-Up
Study." *Arthritis Care & Research* 73, no. 7 (2021): 1041–48.
https://doi.org/10.1002/acr.24220.

Gilpin, Morgan M.; Merritt, Edward; McLean, Scott P.; and Mikan,
Vanessa PhD (2020) "EMG Analysis of Neural Activation Patterns of the Gluteal Muscle Complex," *International Journal of
Exercise Science: Conference Proceedings*: Vol. 2: Iss. 12, Article
165. Available at: https://digitalcommons.wku.edu/ijesab/vol2/
iss12/165.

Hirokawa, S., M. Solomonow, Z. Luo, Y. Lu, and R. D'Ambrosia.
"Muscular Co-Contraction and Control of Knee Stability." *Journal of Electromyography and Kinesiology* 1, no. 3 (1991): 199–208.
https://doi.org/10.1016/1050-6411(91)90035-4.

McGill, Stuart. *Low Back Disorders: Evidence-based Prevention
and Rehabilitation*. Champaign, IL: Human Kinetics, 2007.

Riemann, Bryan L., and Scott M. Lephart. "The Sensorimotor System, Part I: The Physiologic Basis of Functional Joint Stability."
Journal of Athletic Training 37, no. 1 (January 2002): 71–79.

Rombaut, Lies, Fransiska Malfait, Inge De Wandele, Youri Taes,
Youri Thijs, Anne De Paepe, and Patrick Calders. "Muscle
Mass, Muscle Strength, Functional Performance, and Phys-
ical Impairment in Women with the Hypermobility Type of
Ehlers-Danlos Syndrome." *Arthritis Care & Research* 64, no.
10 (2012): 1584–92. https://doi.org/10.1002/acr.21726.

Spinelli, Sam. "Gluteal Amnesia." E3 Rehab. 2019. Accessed January 8, 2022. https://e3rehab.com/blog/glutealamnesia/.

CHAPTER 10: POSTURE

Bates, Alexander Vernon, Alison H. McGregor, and Caroline M. Alexander. "Prolonged Standing Behaviour in People with Joint Hypermobility Syndrome." *BMC Musculoskeletal Disorders* 22, no. 1 (2021): 1005. https://doi.org/10.1186/s12891-021-04744-1.

Booshanam, Divya S., Binu Cherian, Charles Premkumar A. R. Joseph, John Mathew, and Raji Thomas. "Evaluation of Posture and Pain in Persons with Benign Joint Hypermobility Syndrome." *Rheumatology International* 31, no. 12 (2011): 1561–65. https://doi.org/10.1007/s00296-010-1514-2.

Bowman, Katy. *Diastasis Recti*. Calsborg, WA: Propriometrics Press, 2016.

Bowman, Katy. *Move Your DNA*. Carlsborg, WA: Propriometrics Press, 2014.

Claus, Andrew P., Julie A. Hides, G. Lorimer Moseley, and Paul W. Hodges. "Thoracic and Lumbar Posture Behaviour in Sitting Tasks and Standing: Progressing the Biomechanics from Observations to Measurements." *Applied Ergonomics* 53 (2016): 161–68. https://doi.org/10.1016/j.apergo.2015.09.006.

Czaprowski, Dariusz, Paulina Pawłowska, Aleksandra Kolwicz-Gańko, Dominik Sitarski, and Agnieszka Kędra. "The Influence of the 'Straighten Your Back' Command on the Sagittal Spinal Curvatures in Children with Generalized Joint

Hypermobility." *BioMed Research International* 2017 (2017): 1–7. https://doi.org/10.1155/2017/9724021.

Gokhale, Esther. *8 Steps to a Pain-Free Back*. Palo Alto, CA: Pendo Press, 2008.

Greenwood, Naomi L., Lynsey D. Duffell, Caroline M. Alexander, and Alison H. McGregor. "Electromyographic Activity of Pelvic and Lower Limb Muscles during Postural Tasks in People with Benign Joint Hypermobility Syndrome and Non Hypermobile People. A Pilot Study." *Manual Therapy* 16, no. 6 (2011): 623–28. https://doi.org/10.1016/j.math.2011.07.005.

Laird, Robert A., Peter Kent, and Jennifer L. Keating. "How Consistent Are Lordosis, Range of Movement and Lumbo-Pelvic Rhythm in People with and without Back Pain?" *BMC Musculoskeletal Disorders* 17, no. 1 (2016): 403. https://doi.org/10.1186/s12891-016-1250-1.

Preece, Stephen J., Peter Willan, Chris J. Nester, Philip Graham-Smith, Lee Herrington, and Peter Bowker. "Variation in Pelvic Morphology May Prevent the Identification of Anterior Pelvic Tilt." *Journal of Manual & Manipulative Therapy* 16, no. 2 (2008): 113–17. https://doi.org/10.1179/106698108790818459.

Rigoldi, Chiara, Veronica Cimolin, Filippo Camerota, Claudia Celletti, Giorgio Albertini, Luca Mainardi, and Manuela Galli. "Measuring Regularity of Human Postural Sway Using Approximate Entropy and Sample Entropy in Patients with Ehlers-Danlos Syndrome Hypermobility Type." *Research in Developmental Disabilities* 34, no. 2 (2013): 840–46. https://doi.org/10.1016/j.ridd.2012.11.007.

CHAPTER 11: DESIGNING AN ASANA PRACTICE

Coussens, Marie, Bruno Lapauw, Thiberiu Banica, et al. "Muscle Strength, Muscle Mass and Physical Impairment in Women with hypermobile Ehlers-Danlos syndrome and Hypermobility Spectrum Disorder." *Journal of Musculoskeletal and Neuronal Interactions*. Accepted August 23, 2021. http://www.ismni.org/jmni/accepted/JMNI_21M-04-082.pdf.

Cutts, Steven, Mark Prempeh, and Steven Drew. "Anterior Shoulder Dislocation." *The Annals of The Royal College of Surgeons of England* 91, no. 1 (2009): 2–7. https://doi.org/10.1308/003588409X359123.

Desikachar, T.K.V. *The Heart of Yoga*. Rochester, VT: Inner Traditions International Press, 1999.

CHAPTER 12: LANGUAGE AND VERBAL CUES

Eccles, Jessica A., F. D. C. Beacher, M. A. Gray, C. L. Jones, L. Minati, N. A. Harrison, and H. D. Critchley. "Brain Structure and Joint Hypermobility: Relevance to the Expression of Psychiatric Symptoms." *British Journal of Psychiatry* 200, no. 6 (2012): 508–9. https://doi.org/10.1192/bjp.bp.111.092460.

CHAPTER 14: SELF-MASSAGE

Bartsch, Katja Martina, Christian Baumgart, Jürgen Freiwald, Jan Wilke, Gunda Slomka, Sascha Turnhöfer, Christoph Egner, Matthias W. Hoppe, Werner Klingler, and Robert Schleip. "Expert Consensus on the Contraindications and Cautions of Foam Rolling—An International Delphi Study." *Journal of*

Clinical Medicine 10, no. 22 (November 17, 2021): 5360. https://doi.org/10.3390/jcm10225360.

Barreto, Débora M., and Marcus V. A. Batista. "Swedish Massage: A Systematic Review of Its Physical and Psychological Benefits." *Advances in Mind-Body Medicine* 31, no. 2 (Spring 2017): 16–20.

Capobianco, Robyn A., Melissa M. Mazzo, and Roger M. Enoka. "Self-Massage Prior to Stretching Improves Flexibility in Young and Middle-Aged Adults." *Journal of Sports Sciences* 37, no. 13 (July 3, 2019): 1543–50. https://doi.org/10.1080/02640414.2019.1576253.

Ceca, Diego, Laura Elvira, José F. Guzmán, and Ana Pablos. "Benefits of a Self-Myofascial Release Program on Health-Related Quality of Life in People with Fibromyalgia: A Randomized Controlled Trial." *The Journal of Sports Medicine and Physical Fitness* 57, no. 7–8 (August 2017): 993–1002. https://doi.org/10.23736/S0022-4707.17.07025-6.

Cheatham, Scott W., Morey J. Kolber, Matt Cain, and Matt Lee. "The Effects of Self-Myofascial Release Using a Foam Roller or Roller Massager on Joint Range of Motion, Muscle Recovery, and Performance: A Systematic Review." *International Journal of Sports Physical Therapy* 10, no. 6 (November 2015): 827–38.

Clayton, Holly A., Stephanie A. H. Jones, and Denise Y. P. Henriques. "Proprioceptive Precision Is Impaired in Ehlers–Danlos Syndrome." *SpringerPlus* 4, no. 1 (2015): 323. https://doi.org/10.1186/s40064-015-1089-1.

David, Erin, Tal Amasay, Kathryn Ludwig, and Sue Shapiro. "The Effect of Foam Rolling of the Hamstrings on Proprioception at the Knee and Hip Joints." *International Journal of Exercise Science* 12, no. 1 (2019): 343–54.

Hallman, David, and Eugene Lyskov. "Autonomic Regulation in Musculoskeletal Pain." In *Pain in Perspective*, edited by Subhamay Ghosh. InTech, 2012. https://doi.org/10.5772/51086.

Miller, Jill. *The Roll Model: A Step by Step Guide to Erase Pain, Improve Mobility and Live Better in Your Body.* Las Vegas, NV: Victory Belt Publishing, 2014.

Morikawa, Yoshiki, Kouich Takamoto, Hiroshi Nishimaru, Toru Taguchi, Susumu Urakawa, Shigekazu Sakai, Taketoshi Ono, and Hisao Nishijo. "Compression at Myofascial Trigger Point on Chronic Neck Pain Provides Pain Relief through the Prefrontal Cortex and Autonomic Nervous System: A Pilot Study." *Frontiers in Neuroscience* 11 (April 11, 2017). https://doi.org/10.3389/fnins.2017.00186.

Kovaleva, L.A., and V.V. Kovalev. "Justification of the Effectiveness of the Technique of Myofascial Self-Massage Using Tennis Balls in Fitness." *Health, Sport, Rehabilitation* 5, no. 3 (October 14, 2019): 53. https://doi.org/10.34142/HSR.2019.05.03.06.

Schroeder, Allison N., and Thomas M. Best. "Is Self-Myofascial Release an Effective Preexercise and Recovery Strategy? A Literature Review." *Current Sports Medicine Reports* 14, no. 3 (2015): 200–208. https://doi.org/10.1249/JSR.0000000000000148.

Shin, Mal-Soon, and Yun-Hee Sung. "Effects of Massage on Muscular Strength and Proprioception after Exercise-Induced Muscle Damage." *Journal of Strength and Conditioning Research* 29, no. 8 (August 2015): 2255–60. https://doi.org/10.1519/JSC.0000000000000688.

Soares, Rogerio N., Erin Calaine Inglis, Rojan Khoshreza, Juan M. Murias, and Saied Jalal Aboodarda. "Rolling Massage Acutely Improves Skeletal Muscle Oxygenation and Parameters Associated with Microvascular Reactivity: The First Evidence-Based Study." *Microvascular Research* 132 (2020): 104063. https://doi.org/10.1016/j.mvr.2020.104063.

Wiewelhove, Thimo, Alexander Döweling, Christoph Schneider, Laura Hottenrott, Tim Meyer, Michael Kellmann, Mark Pfeiffer, and Alexander Ferrauti. "A Meta-Analysis of the Effects of Foam Rolling on Performance and Recovery." *Frontiers in Physiology* 10 (April 9, 2019): 376. https://doi.org/10.3389/fphys.2019.00376.

CHAPTER 15: CALMING THE NERVOUS SYSTEM

Alshak, Mark N., and Joe M. Das. "Neuroanatomy, Sympathetic Nervous System." In *StatPearls*. Treasure Island (FL): StatPearls Publishing, 2022. http://www.ncbi.nlm.nih.gov/books/NBK542195/.

Bodison, Stefanie C., and L. Diane Parham. "Specific Sensory Techniques and Sensory Environmental Modifications for Children and Youth With Sensory Integration Difficulties: A Systematic Review." *The American Journal of Occupational*

Therapy 72, no. 1 (January 1, 2018): 7201190040p1–11. https://doi.org/10.5014/ajot.2018.029413.

Bonaz, B., V. Sinniger, and S. Pellissier. "Vagal Tone: Effects on Sensitivity, Motility, and Inflammation." *Neurogastroenterology & Motility* 28, no. 4 (2016): 455–62. https://doi.org/10.1111/nmo.12817.

Dana, Deb. *The Polyvagal Theory in Therapy: Engaging the Rhythm of Regulation*. New York: W. W. Norton & Company, 2018.

Kolacz, Jacek, Katja Kovacic, Gregory F. Lewis, Manu R. Sood, Qasim Aziz, Olivia R. Roath, and Stephen W. Porges. "Cardiac Autonomic Regulation and Joint Hypermobility in Adolescents with Functional Abdominal Pain Disorders." *Neurogastroenterology & Motility* 33, no. 12 (2021). https://doi.org/10.1111/nmo.14165.

Kovacic, Katja, Jacek Kolacz, Gregory F. Lewis, and Stephen W. Porges. "Impaired Vagal Efficiency Predicts Auricular Neurostimulation Response in Adolescent Functional Abdominal Pain Disorders." *American Journal of Gastroenterology* 115, no. 9 (2020): 1534–38. https://doi.org/10.14309/ajg.0000000000000753.

Laborde, Sylvain, Emma Mosley, and Julian F. Thayer. "Heart Rate Variability and Cardiac Vagal Tone in Psychophysiological Research–Recommendations for Experiment Planning, Data Analysis, and Data Reporting." *Frontiers in Psychology* 08 (February 20, 2017). https://doi.org/10.3389/fpsyg.2017.00213.

Porges, Stephen W. "Orienting in a Defensive World: Mammalian Modifications of Our Evolutionary Heritage. A Polyvagal Theory." *Psychophysiology* 32, no. 4 (1995): 301–18. https://doi.org/10.1111/j.1469-8986.1995.tb01213.x.

Porges, Stephen W. "The Polyvagal Theory: New Insights into Adaptive Reactions of the Autonomic Nervous System." *Cleveland Clinic Journal of Medicine* 76, no. 4 suppl 2 (2009): S86–90. https://doi.org/10.3949/ccjm.76.s2.17.

Porges, Stephen W. *The Pocket Guide to The Polyvagal Theory: The Transformative Power of Feeling Safe.* New York: W. W. Norton & Company, Inc., 2017.

Reynolds, Stacey, Shelly J. Lane, and Brian Mullen. "Effects of Deep Pressure Stimulation on Physiological Arousal." *The American Journal of Occupational Therapy* 69, no. 3 (May 1, 2015): 6903350010p1–5. https://doi.org/10.5014/ajot.2015.015560.

Rosenberg, Stanley. *Accessing the Healing Power of the Vagus Nerve.* California: North Atlantic Books, 2017.

CHAPTER 16: FOCUSING THE MIND

Daubenmier, Jennifer, Jocelyn Sze, Catherine E. Kerr, Margaret E. Kemeny, and Wolf Mehling. "Follow Your Breath: Respiratory Interoceptive Accuracy in Experienced Meditators: Respiratory Interoceptive Accuracy in Meditators." *Psychophysiology* 50, no. 8 (2013): 777–89. https://doi.org/10.1111/psyp.12057.

Froeliger, Brett, Eric L. Garland, and F. Joseph McClernon. "Yoga Meditation Practitioners Exhibit Greater Gray Matter Volume and Fewer Reported Cognitive Failures: Results of a Preliminary Voxel-Based Morphometric Analysis." *Evidence-Based Complementary and Alternative Medicine* 2012 (2012): 1–8. https://doi.org/10.1155/2012/821307.

Glans, Martin, Nils Thelin, Mats B. Humble, Marie Elwin, and Susanne Bejerot. "Association between Adult Attention-Deficit Hyperactivity Disorder and Generalised Joint Hypermobility: A Cross-Sectional Case Control Comparison." *Journal of Psychiatric Research* 143 (2021): 334–40. https://doi.org/10.1016/j.jpsychires.2021.07.006.

Gothe, Neha, Matthew B. Pontifex, Charles Hillman, and Edward McAuley. "The Acute Effects of Yoga on Executive Function." *Journal of Physical Activity and Health* 10, no. 4 (2013): 488–95. https://doi.org/10.1123/jpah.10.4.488.

Gothe, Neha P., Jessica M. Hayes, Cindy Temali, and Jessica S. Damoiseaux. "Differences in Brain Structure and Function Among Yoga Practitioners and Controls." *Frontiers in Integrative Neuroscience* 12 (June 22, 2018): 26. https://doi.org/10.3389/fnint.2018.00026.

Mitchell, John T., Elizabeth M. McIntyre, Joseph S. English, Michelle F. Dennis, Jean C. Beckham, and Scott H. Kollins. "A Pilot Trial of Mindfulness Meditation Training for ADHD in Adulthood: Impact on Core Symptoms, Executive Functioning, and Emotion Dysregulation." *Journal of Attention Disorders* 21, no. 13 (2017): 1105–20. https://doi.org/10.1177/1087054713513328.

Printed in Great Britain
by Amazon